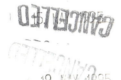

VIRUSES
AND
IMMUNITY

ACADEMIC PRESS RAPID MANUSCRIPT REPRODUCTION

VIRUSES
AND
IMMUNITY

Toward Understanding Viral Immunology
and Immunopathology

Edited by

Claude Koprowski

Downstate Medical College
Brooklyn, New York

Hilary Koprowski

The Wistar Institute
of Anatomy and Biology
Philadelphia, Pennsylvania

Academic Press, Inc.   New York   San Francisco   London   1975
A Subsidiary of Harcourt Brace Jovanovich, Publishers

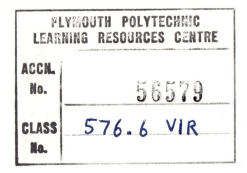
ACADEMIC PRESS, INC.
111 Fifth Avenue, New York, New York 10003

United Kingdom Edition published by
ACADEMIC PRESS, INC. (LONDON) LTD.
24/28 Oval Road, London NW1

Library of Congress Cataloging in Publication Data
Main entry under title:

Viruses and immunity.

    Consists of material which was presented at a series
of interinstitutional seminars organized by the Wistar
Institute of Anatomy and Biology, Philadelphia, and the
Graduate Group in Immunology, University of Pennsylvania,
in 1973, and revised prior to publication.
    Bibliography: p.
    Includes index.
    1.   Virus diseases—Immunological aspects—Congresses.
I. Koprowski, Claude, ed.   II.   Koprowski, Hilary, ed.
[DNLM: 1.   Virus diseases—Immunology—Congresses.
2.   Viruses—Immunology—Congresses.   QW160 V8212 1973]
RC114.5.V48   616.01'94   75-1473
ISBN 0–12–420350–7

CONTENTS

LIST OF CONTRIBUTORS

Herman Friedman, Department of Microbiology, Albert Einstein Medical Center, Philadelphia, Pennsylvania 19141

Donald H. Gilden, The Wistar Institute of Anatomy and Biology, Philadelphia, Pennsylvania 19104

Diane Griffin, Department of Neurology, The Johns Hopkins University School of Medicine, Baltimore, Maryland 21205

Abner L. Notkins, National Institute of Dental Research, National Institutes of Health, Bethesda, Maryland 20014

Stanley A. Plotkin, The Wistar Institute of Anatomy and Biology, Philadelphia, Pennsylvania 19104

Richmond T. Prehn, The Institute for Cancer Research, Philadelphia, Pennsylvania 19111

Frantisek Sokol, The Wistar Institute of Anatomy and Biology, Philadelphia, Pennsylvania 19104

Alfred D. Steinberg, Arthritis and Rheumatism Branch, NIAMD; National Institutes of Health, Bethesda, Maryland 20014

Osias Stutman, Sloan Kettering Institute for Cancer Research, New York, New York 10021

E. Frederick Wheelock, Department of Microbiology, Jefferson Medical College of Thomas Jefferson University, Philadelphia, Pennsylvania 19107

PREFACE

In the explosive field of immunology it has been difficult to keep abreast of developments in viral immunology and viral immunopathology. Part of the problem stems from the small number of researchers specializing in this area; part from the limited training that has been available in the field; and part from the circumscribed coverage given it in general texts.

It was with these thoughts in mind that The Wistar Institute of Anatomy and Biology, Philadelphia, and the Graduate Group in Immunology at the University of Pennsylvania organized a series of interinstitutional seminars. Their goal was to survey the current state of knowledge in viral immunology and immunopathology and to discuss selected *basic* findings which could serve as an ancilla for further understanding and future experimental work.

These seminars met with such interest that it was decided to organize the material presented for publication. Although the seminars were given in 1973, the principal participants had the opportunity to revise their contributions just prior to publication so the material covered is as recent as production schedules would allow.

Viruses and Immunity: Toward Understanding Viral Immunology and Immunopathology covers a number of basic concepts dealing with immunodeficiency states and experimental immunosuppression. It looks at the immune responses in tumor growth and the role of immune complexes and autoimmune phenomena in virus infections. Finally, it covers current concepts of viral immunoprophylaxis and immunotherapy.

No attempt has been made to treat the subject matter panoramically in textbook fashion. We feel that in a field which, like *Six Characters in Search of an Author,* is still awaiting a unifying genius, an attempt at a uniform view would be contrary to the reader's best interests. Rather, the participants and editors have attempted to examine highly selected areas in depth. The reader will note that authors offer a rich diversity of views, some of them treating similar experimental data from highly varied perspectives with equally varied interpretations.

Although the authors cover a number of basic ideas, this book is not aimed at readers without a general grasp of immunology and virology. Those who gleaned the most from the seminars were junior and senior medical students, clinicians who have kept abreast of general developments in immunology and ·for whom clinical examples have been included wherever practical, and graduate students of microbiology and immunology. As the text was designed for fairly rapid reading, abundant references have been included for those who wish to pursue the matter covered either more universally or in greater depth.

We are especially grateful to Mrs. Lorraine A. DiLorenzo for her preparation of the manuscripts and correspondence with the contributors, and to Mrs. Evelyn H. Webb for her assistance in proofreading the material.

Claude Koprowski
Hilary Koprowski

INTRODUCTORY REMARKS

Abner Louis Notkins

Laboratory of Oral Medicine
National Institute of Dental Research
National Institutes of Health
Bethesda, Maryland

Over the last five years there has been a renewal of interest in the manner by which the host defends itself against viral infections. This stems from several important developments. First, it has been shown that a number of viruses can persist in the host for months or years, despite the presence of neutralizing antibody. Examples of persistent infections in man are herpes simplex virus (HSV), cytomegalovirus, Epstein-Barr virus, hepatitis B virus, wart virus, and the agents that produce subacute sclerosing panencephalitis and progressive multifocal leukoencephalopathy. In animals, viruses such as lactic dehydrogenase, lymphocytic choriomeningitis (LCM) murine leukemia, Aleutian disease, equine infectious anemia, Marek's disease and SV-40 can all produce persistent infections. Second, there is now good evidence indicating that cellular immunity may be a crucial determinant in stopping the spread of certain viral infections such as HSV. Third, experiments from a number of laboratories have shown that under certain circumstances the immune response to a viral infection, rather than the destructive capacity of the virus itself, may be responsible for the clinical and pathologic manifestations of the infection.

How the immune response of the host stops viral infections appears to be intimately related to the mode by which the virus spreads. Basically viruses can spread by three different routes; extracellularly (Type I spread); from cell-to-contiguous cell (Type II spread); or from parent to progeny cell during cell division (Type III spread). An example of Type I spread is poliovirus; Type II, HSV; and Type III, the murine leukemia viruses or SV-40. A number of viruses, however, can spread by more than one route; HSV, for example, spreads by both the Type I and II routes.

It is becoming quite clear that different immunological processes are required to stop the different modes of viral spread. Type I spread is usually stopped by the neutralization of extracellular virus by antiviral antibody. The initial step in neutralization is the attachment of antibody to the virus, but if the amount of antibody bound to the virus is small or if the antibody is not attached to "critical sites" the result may not be neutralization, but the formation of infectious virus-antibody complexes. Only when larger amounts of antibody attach to the virus, and attach in the right place, does neutralization occur. Neutralization may occur either before the virus reaches the cell or at the level of the cell itself. Before the virus reaches the cell, antibody may neutralize the virus either by aggregating virus particles and thereby reducing the number of infectious units or by lysing the virion with the aid of complement. At the level of the cell, antibody may neutralize the virus by covering the surface of the virion thereby preventing attachment, penetration or uncoating. If antibody alone fails to neutralize the virus, the host has available to it certain accessory factors such as complement and rheumatoid factor, which may enhance the amount of neutralization produced by the antibody.

The class of the immunoglobulin involved in viral neutralization depends on the site of the infection. IgA antibody secreted by the mucous surfaces of the body is the first line of defense localizing the infection to the epithelial surfaces. IgA is therefore particularly important in combating infections of the respiratory and digestive tracts. If the virus gets into the blood, the predominant immunoglobulins in the blood, IgG and IgM, come into action, neutralizing the virus with or without the help of complement and other accessory factors.

How the host stops Type II spread is even more complex. In this case the virus is protected from neutralizing antibody because it is able to spread from cell-to-contiguous cell as a result of virus-induced cell fusion. If, however, the virus induces new antigens on the surface of the infected cell, recognition of these antigens by specific antiviral antibody and complement or immune lymphocytes can result in cell destruction. This would stop the spread of the virus provided the destruction of the infected cell occurred before the virus had spread to adjacent uninfected cells. If, however, the infected cell was destroyed after the virus had spread, the infection would not be stopped. Under these conditions, the host might still stop the spread of the infection by intervening at the junction between infected and uninfected cells or by acting on uninfected cells. For example, inflammatory cells attracted to the site of the infection might be "toxic" on a nonspecific basis to both infected and uninfected cells and thereby hinder virus-induced cell fusion. This could convert a Type II into a Type I spread; the latter can be effectively handled by the simple neutralization of extracellular virus. Alternatively, immune lymphocytes stimulated by viral antigens can release readily diffusable biological mediators such as chemotactic factors, lymphotoxin, and interferon. The latter could prevent uninfected cells at the site of the lesion from becoming infected. From *in vitro* studies, it is known that interferon released from a relatively small number of lymphocytes can protect a large number of target cells. Thus, cell-mediated immunity appears to operate, in part, through the release of interferon. Although most cells of the body are capable of making interferon, certain viruses are poor interferon inducers. The cell-mediated immune response may be particularly important against these viruses in that it amplifies the host's interferon-producing capacity at the site of the local infection.

How the host stops Type III spread is even less clearly understood. Viruses that spread by this route are often nonlytic; the viral genome may be integrated into the host-cell genome and during cell division the viral genome is passed on to progeny cells. To stop Type III spread it is necessary either to destroy the infected cell or to stop cell division. Whether the immune response is successful in destroying the infected cell depends in part upon whether or not the virus induces a sufficient amount of new antigens on the surface of the cell so that the cell is recognized as foreign by immune lymphocytes or by antibody and complement.

Information as to the relative importance of humoral versus cellular immunity in combating a particular viral infection has been obtained from patients with specific immunological deficiencies and from animals by (*a*) selective suppression of either the cellular or humoral components of the immune system(e. g., thymectomy or bursectomy); or (*b*) passive administration of immune cells or serum to virus-infected animals. Although data are still far from complete, these studies support the idea that humoral immunity is needed to stop those viruses which spread by the extracellular route (Type I), whereas cell-mediated immunity plays an important role in stopping viruses that spread from cell-to-contiguous cell (Type II). When, however, the immunologically uncompromised host is infected, the whole army of weapons appears to be mobilized, i.e., antibody is made and lymphocytes are stimulated. Which defense mechanism actually stops the infection then depends on the mode of viral spread. The various weapons are mobilized because the host does not know which type of spread the virus will actually use and it tries to prepare itself for all of them.

The immune response to a viral infection, however, is not always beneficial to the host. In the case of acute LCM infection in adult mice, the virus itself produces little injury. It is the host's immune response to virus-infected cells which is responsible for cell destruction and the subsequent death of the animal. In the case of chronic LCM infection, the interaction of antibody with viral antigens leads to the deposition of virus-antibody complexes in the kidneys, and this results in the development of glomerulonephritis. The possibility that immune complexes of viral origin may be involved in the pathogenesis of human glomerulonephritis is now being investigated in several laboratories.

Why so many viruses persist in the presence of immunity remains a challenging and still unresolved problem. A number of reasons can be cited and others can be postulated. In the case of HSV, for example, the virus remains latent in sensory ganglia for years where it appears to be antigenically invisible, but capable of being reactivated by a number of factors including nerve injury. In certain infections, such as with lactic dehydrogenase virus, the interaction of antibody with the virus may fail to neutralize the virus, resulting in the formation of infectious virus-antibody complexes. Other viruses, such as the leukemia viruses can infect the cells of the immune system and thereby depress the immune response of the host. In still other cases, the destruction of virus-infected cells by specifically immune lymphocytes can sometimes be blocked at the level of the target cells by the binding of anti-viral antibody or at the level of the lymphocyte by immune complexes.

Persistent viral infections cause considerable morbidity and mortality in both animals and man. Is it going to be possible to develop effective vaccines against viruses that produce persistent infections? Is there any way of curing individuals once they become chronically infected? If, for example, lack of antigenic expression on the cell surface underlies the persistence of certain viral infections, then attempts to stimulate the immune system may not be useful. Under these circumstances nonimmunological factors, such as chemotherapy or interferon, may be required. In still other cases, where the immune response to the virus is responsible for the disease, immunosuppression may prove to be the treatment of choice. Methods of preventing and treating persistent viral infections appear to represent one of the great challenges of the future in the field of viral immunology.

1

Immunodeficiency States and Natural Resistance

Osias Stutman

We assume that natural resistance to the "infectious"
world within and around us is mediated by immune mechanisms.
Thus, any deficiency of the immune system will lead to a decrease of natural resistance to infections. The validity of
such an assumption is based on the increased susceptibility
to infections observed in animals and man as a result of
spontaneous or induced immune deficiencies.

Immunological reactions are complex mixtures of specific
and non-specific effects interacting in a delicate balance.
These components are: 1. antibody-mediated reactions;
2. cell-mediated reactions (mainly thymus-dependent) and
3. other effector mechanisms which include phagocytosis by
granular and mononuclear phagocytes (leukocytes, circulating
and fixed histiocytes, etc.) and the small vessel reactions
mediated by smooth muscle contraction, inflammation and blood
coagulation. There are also biological amplification systems
which include: a. the classical activation of the complement system by the interaction of antigen with antibody;
b. the alternate pathway of complement activation by a wide
variety of mechanisms (endotoxin, proteolytic enzymes, coagulation factors, etc); c. the kinin system of vasoactive
substances and d. the production by lymphocytes and other
cells of a large number of biologically active substances
(lymphokines) capable of acting on mitotic rates, cell metabolism, cell motility and cell function. From the interactions of these factors, integrated responses occur, which
most probably represent our basic defense mechanisms against
infections (see reference 1 for a review of these interactions). We will concentrate our discussion on analyzing the
role of some of such factors (antibodies, cell-mediated

immunity with special emphasis on the role of thymus) and the overall resistance-susceptibility to infections and malignancy.

IMMUNODEFICIENCY STATES AND INFECTIONS

The definition and characterization of different immunodeficiency syndromes in man has permitted an interesting approach to the study of infections. All forms of primary immunodeficiency in man are accompanied by an increased susceptibility to infections (2). The interesting fact is that the pathogenic agents are quite different when the various syndromes are compared (2). In the humoral immune deficiency syndrome, of which the sex-linked recessive form of agammaglobulinemia (Bruton's) is the prototype (3), the most common infections are pneumonitis, meningitis, otitis, etc. The common agents in these cases are mainly the high-grade encapsulated pyogenic pathogens (pneumococcus, streptococcus, meningococcus) as well as haemophilus influenza and pseudomonas aeruginosa (2,4). Agammaglobulinemic patients have also an increased susceptibility to hepatitis, developing a fulminating type of infection (5). In the cell-mediated immune deficiency syndrome, of which the congenital absence of the thymus and parathyroids (DiGeorge's syndrome) is the prototype (6,7) as well as in the combined deficiencies of which the thymic displasia or Swiss-type lymphopenic agammaglobulinemia (8) and the sex-linked lymphopenic immunologic deficiency (9,10) are the best examples, the infectious picture is quite different (2). These patients suffer severe and often lethal viral infections (rubeola, varicella, cytomegalic inclusion virus) and smallpox vaccination may lead to progressive vaccinia (2,11). They also suffer from severe fungal infections especially with candida albicans and histoplasma capsulatum (2) and they may have fatal generalized reactions to Bacillus Calmette-Gerin (BCG) vaccination (2,12). Also chronic pulmonary infections with low pathogenic agents such as Pneumocystis Carinii are common complications (13). Many of these infections are life threatening and represent the major clinical problem in the management of these patients (2,10). Similarly, these types of infections are common complications of induced immunosuppression in patients treated for kidney transplants (14,15). In the 9th Report of the Human Renal Transplantation Registry, sepsis accounted for the highest cause of death (30%) in renal allograft recipients (16). It is apparent that immunologic deficiencies in man whether spontaneous or induced, whether partial or total, are accompanied by an inordinate frequency of infections (2).

2

Isolated IgA deficiency is associated with a high incidence of sinopulmonary infections, intestinal malabsorption and/or sprue-like syndromes and a variety of autoimmune diseases (17). The Wiskott-Aldrich syndrome is a complex disease that includes abnormalities of platelet function as well as immune inadequacy, especially deficient in responses to polysaccharide antigens (18,19). These children also suffer from recurring, life threatening infections of lungs, skin and other tissues and may have overwhelming disease with herpes simplex, varicella or pneumocystis carinii (18). Similarly, patients with ataxia-telangiectasia, which is a complex disease that includes a combined immune deficiency of both cellular and humoral responses, are also plagued with multiple infections, especially sinopulmonary infections (20). The late-onset (acquired) hypogammaglobulinemia, which includes a number of different diseases such as sporadic agammaglobulinemia, the various types of dysgammaglobulinemias, the so-called acquired agammaglobulinemias and the primary immunologic deficiency of adults, are the most common types of immune deficiency in man (21). These diseases are also characterized by a high incidence of infections especially with encapsulated pyogenic extracellular pathogens (21) and by an inordinate incidence of autoimmune diseases (22). For a more detailed analysis of the association of autoimmunity with immune deficiency diseases see reference 23 and Chapter 8.

Deficiencies of the amplification systems or of leukocyte bactericidal capacity are also associated with an increased incidence of infections. A few examples of this are: a) deficiencies related to C3, a complement component, are associated with recurrent pneumonias (24); b) a deficit of Clr, another complement component, leads to increased frequency of infections and vasculitis (25); c) similarly a deficiency of C2 is accompanied by an increased incidence of infections (26); (for a complete review of complement deficiencies in humans and increased incidence of infections, kidney disease and autoimmunity see reference 27); d) the defect known as chronic granulomatous disease in which leukocytes are capable of phagocytosis although they cannot destroy the ingested bacteria (28,29) is also accompanied by an increased susceptibility to infections.

Therefore, it is quite apparent from the clinical data that a close link exists between an intact immune system and the capacity to deal effectively with bacterial, viral or fungal infections.

The experimental evidence between the association of an intact immune system with susceptibility to infections is compelling. For example, neonatally thymectomized mice are more susceptible than sham-operated controls to infections with hepatotropic viruses (30,31), herpes simplex virus (32), mycobacterium leprae (33), Candida albicans (34), the endotoxins of Escherichia Coli and Salmonella Typhosa (34), to infections with Leishmania (35), Trypanosoma (36), Plasmodium (37), other nematodes in rats (38), schistosoma (39), etc. These effects have been described not only in mice and rats but also in other species such as chickens and rabbits.

In some instances, the effects of thymectomy are somewhat paradoxical since by eliminating the cell-mediated response they do eliminate a pathogenic factor of the clinical disease, and as is the case with the lympho-chorio-meningitis virus, the actual cause of death (40). A somewhat similar reaction occurs with Leishmania infections in mice, in which there is a delay in the appearance of the lesions, although the infection is more severe (35).

Two anecdotes help show the link between an intact immune system and susceptibility to infections:

In his original description of the nude trait in mice, Flanagan defined the genetics of such a trait and had to accept that it was a single locus producing multiple genetic defects which included poor hair development and a liver disease which caused early death (41). Flanagan indicated that the hepatic lesions could be metabolic but that all the nude mice showed granulomas suggesting Toxoplasma Gondii infection (41). Approximately two years later it was discovered that the nude mice also had an absence of thymic development (42), which explained the liver lesion only in the homozygote nu/nu and not in the heterozygote nu/+ (which have a normal thymus)as a result of the presence of Toxoplasma as an endemic parasite in the colony associated with the profound immune deficiency in such mice.

In 1896 Abelous and Billard thymectomized frogs and observed that all the animals died by the 14th day after the operation with a disease characterized by muscular weakness and later paralysis, loss of normal skin color, skin ulcers, progressive anemia, leucocytosis, hemorraghic lesions, edema and death (43). If only the thymic lobe was removed, such symptoms did not occur and blood from such sick animals could produce the same symptoms when injected into normal animals (43). The authors interpreted their results as an indication that the thymus elaborates substances which neutralize toxins formed during normal metabolism and that the thymus is "an essential organ for life" (43). Three years

4

later, Ver Eecke thymectomized frogs and observed that the symptoms reported by Abelous and Billard did not occur if the water in the tanks was changed frequently, but developed only when the water was allowed to stagnate (44). Ver Eecke's conclusions were that the pathologic condition observed after thymectomy resulted from infections fostered by contaminated water and not from absence of the thymus (44). In 1905 Hammar was unable to reproduce Abelous and Billard experiments, using only clean animals (45). Finally, Pari isolated an organism, a bacillus resembling the one producing gangrenous septicemia, from the blood and organs of thymectomized frogs that were sick after confinement in unchanged waters (46,47). He succeeded in producing the disease in both thymectomized and normal frogs by direct inoculation of the agent; however, he observed that the disease was severe, generalized and lethal in the thymectomized frogs while it was usually localized to the injection site and rarely fatal in the sham-thymectomized controls (46,47). Pari's interpretation was that the loss of the thymus rendered the animals more susceptible to the particular infection described and "probably to all infections" (46,47). This was, indeed, the first statement on a direct relationship between thymus function and immunity. This lead was not followed, and for the next 50 years the work on the thymus followed the conventional endocrinologic pathway, attempting to demonstrate all kinds of hormonal functions. Incidentally, thymectomy of frog larvae produces the same immune deficiencies as those observed in mammals (48).

Other fragments of evidence from the clinic also indicate that the spleen is important in resistance to infections: splenectomized children and those with congenital asplenia show an undue susceptibility to severe and frequently fatal pneumococcal sepsis (49), and splenectomized rats have impaired clearing of pneumococcus from blood (50).

It is apparent that an intact immune system is a requirement for adequate handling of a wide variety of infectious agents. It is in this context that Ehrlich wrote in 1909 that "Fortunately, these germs (keime) remain inactive in the majority of the people because of the immune system" (51). In that same article Ehrlich added that: "If this self protection did not exist we could expect that carcinomas would appear with overwhelming frequency" (51), which brings us directly to our next subject.

IMMUNODEFICIENCY STATES AND MALIGNANCY

Ehrlich was indeed the first to suggest the possibility
of the immune system to act as a defense mechanism against
malignancy (51). Fifty years later, Thomas proposed that the
justification for cell-mediated immunity could be, among
other functions, to deal with malignant cells (52). Thomas
wrote that because of the "...universal requirement of multi-
cellular organisms to preserve uniformity of cell·type...
homograft rejection will turn out to represent a primary
mechanism for natural defense against neoplasia" (52). This
originated as an attempt to justify the presence of a system
that was capable of dealing very efficiently with surgical
artifacts such as transplants. An alternative explanation
was that "...the homograft reaction may be regarded as the
price paid for an efficient system of defense against bacterial and viral invasion" (53). As was indicated in a
review: "The ability to reject foreign transplants is so
consistent in phylogeny that it must represent an important
survival advantage to the species endowed with it, an advantage that has no relation to modern organ transplantation"
(54).

The possible role of immune functions controlling in some
way the development of malignant tumors became crystallized
in the theory of "immune surveillance" (55,56), the evolu-
tionary significance of which is preventing the emergence of
malignant mutant cells (55). The association of spontaneous
or induced immune deficiency with increased incidence of
tumors, both in experimental animals and man, has been indicated as supportive evidence of the immune surveillance
theory (57,58).

This immune surveillance theory is supported by three
types of evidence: a) the effects of immunosuppression in
experimental animals, which according to the dogma should
"foster malignant development" (56,58); b) the malignancies
appearing in immunodepressed patients (59) and c) the apparent high incidence of malignancy in patients with different
immunodeficiency diseases (58).

The data with experimental animals, briefly summarized,
indicates that the issue is not simple, and probably that
immune surveillance may not be an all-pervading generalized
phenomenon but a more restricted event (see reference 60 for
review). It is agreed that immunosuppression, either as
thymectomy or treatment with anti-lymphocyte serum, has a
clear effect on increasing tumor incidence after polyoma
virus infection (61,62), other DNA oncogenic viruses (63,64),
herpes-type (Marek) virus (65) and Moloney-sarcoma virus

(66,67). In the last instance, we have observed that in
nude athymic adult BALB/C mice infected with Moloney-sarcoma virus, the overall incidence of tumors is similar to
that observed in normal BALB/C mice, but the tumors do not
regress in the nude athymic mice (67). On the other hand,
immunodepression has only limited effects on the erythroid
malignancy induced by Friend leukemia virus in mice (68).
We have observed that, depending on the genetic makeup of
the different strains, such animals could be divided into
two groups of resistant strains: those which became sensitive after immunodepression and those that remained resistant after effective immunodepression (68).

With chemical carcinogens the issue is even more complex.
For studies using mainly polycyclic hydrocarbons the results
indicate that thymectomy increases tumor incidence (69,70,
71,72) or has no detectable effect (73,74,75 and Stutman,
unpublished). The same discrepancies with effects of anti-
lymphocyte serum or similar preparations: increase in tumor
incidence and/or decrease in latency periods were described
(76,77,78) as well as no detectable effects (79,80,81,82).
On the other hand, we have observed that tumor incidence
after methylcholanthrene was comparable in every possible
parameter between nude athymic mice, which have a profound
immune deficit,and their normal heterozygote brothers (83).
Higher incidence of lung adenomas after urethan has been
described in thymectomized mice (84); however, we could not
observe such an increase in lung adenomas either after
methylcholanthrene or urethan in nude athymic mice (67,83).
Similarly, the incidence of spontaneous tumors in animals
subjected to chronic immunosuppression by anti-lymphocyte
serum is not increased (81,82). In the athymic nude mouse,
the incidence of spontaneous tumors is either comparable to
that observed in normal mice of the same age and strain, or
slightly decreased (67,83,85,86). It is apparent that in
many of these mouse experiments some of the discrepancies
could be derived from differences in animal care or strains.
However, they do not form such a strong support for the idea
of a generalized immune surveillance defense mechanism, but
more of a restricted phenomenon that applies only to certain
malignancies.

The high incidence of primary malignancies appearing in
patients that are chronically immunosuppressed for organ
transplantation needs clarification (59,87). The latest
figures indicate that organ transplant recipients maintained
on chronic immunosuppressive therapy have a 5-6% chance of
developing a de novo malignant tumor within the first few
years after transplantation (59). There are approximately

7

122 such cases from different transplant centers (59) for
a population at a risk of approximately 3,000 patients (16).
Of such tumors, 61% were of epithelial origin and 38% were
mesenchimal (59). The most common epithelial lesions were
various skin cancers (27 cases, 36%), carcinomas of the cer-
vix (11 cases, 14%) and carcinoma of the lip (11 cases, 14%).
The remainder were different types of visceral tumors, some
of high malignancy (59). Of the 49 (38%) mesenchimal tumors,
42 (86%) were solid lymphomas of which the most common sub-
group was reticulum cell sarcoma (30 cases). A most unusual feature of the lymphomas was their predilection for the
central nervous system (20 of 42 cases) (59). Some discrepancies, i.e., higher incidence of mesenchimal tumors in
the 42 cases reported from different centers (21 cases with
mesenchimal tumors) versus only 3 of 15 (20%) for the series
at the University of Colorado (87), were explained as "a
reporting artifact in that there would be a tendency to report only the more florid and lethal malignancies to the
registry" (87). The importance of the epithelial tumors appearing in the immunosuppressed patients in relation to immune surveillance is that probably they cannot be attributed
to a direct effect of the immunosuppressive drugs. Such
criticism has been raised against the mesenchimal tumors and
lymphomas appearing in the immunosuppressed patients (88).
On the other hand, the appearance of malignancies in other
types of patients under chronic immunosuppressive therapy
is not well documented, although a recent review indicates
that chemically immunosuppressed humans receiving organ
transplants are more likely to develop lymphoreticular
tumors than those without organ transplants (89). However,
an apparent increase in the incidence of skin cancers has
been observed in patients with psoriasis under chronic
immunosuppression (90).

Chronic antigenic stimulation has produced an increased
incidence of reticular tumors in mice (91) and these effects
are increased when chronic antigenic stimulation is associated with chemical immunosuppression (92). It is apparent
that such possibilities could be important factors in ex-
plaining high lymphoma incidences in the immunosuppressed
organ recipients and the chronically infected humans with
primary immunodeficiencies. However, when this hypothesis
was tested in a most elegant epidemiologic study, the results
did not support the association of immunosuppression plus
chronic antigenic stimulation with either higher incidence of
cancers or of leukemia-lymphoma(93). In this study, a large
number of patients with leprosy, including sufficient numbers
of lepromatous and tuberculoid leprosy, were analyzed for

overall incidence of malignant disease and of leukemia-lymphoma (93). The rationale behind these studies was that the leprosy patients have a defect of cell-mediated immunity and are also submitted to chronic antigenic stimulation and the results indicated that based on person-years-at-risk analysis and age, sex, race and calendar-specific U.S. cancer mortality rates, there were no differences in the observed and expected incidence of tumors or leukemia-lymphoma cases in such patients (93).

The main problem with the association of certain diseases with high incidence of malignancy is in many instances one of an epidemiological analysis of the cases. For example, the association of high incidence of lymphoma-leukemia with certain autoimmune diseases, did not resist analysis when a large number of case reports were compiled and compared with adequate controls for tumor risk (94,95). Similar results were obtained by the retrospective analysis of antecedent autoimmune disease among children with leukemia-lymphoma and it was apparent from such studies that there were no differences in incidence of autoimmunity either in the propositi or family members when compared with matched controls (96). Thus, many of these "anecdotes" concerning interesting associations of malignancy with other primary diseases are still open to further analysis. The main problem, indicated in one of the above cited papers (94) is that "case reports are known to be subject to a myriad of selection biases..." This remark brings us directly to the high incidence of malignancies in patients with primary immunodeficiencies (97,98,99,100).

Data from a newly established Immunodeficiency-Cancer Registry (99) shows 151 tumors in 145 patients with primary immunodeficiency syndromes, including: sex-linked (Bruton's) agammaglobulinemia, 6 patients; severe combined system immunodeficiency, 9 patients; Wiskott-Aldrich syndrome, 24 patients;ataxia-telangiectasia, 52 patients; common variable (late onset) immunodeficiency, 41 patients; isolated IgA deficiency, 7 patients and isolated IgM deficiency, 6 patients. For the total group the incidence and type of tumors was 58% lymphoreticular, 17% leukemias, 18% epithelial, 3% mesenchimal and 4% involving the nervous system (99). The latest figures including now 163 patients show that still the incidence of lymphoreticular tumors is 57% and that of leukemias is 17% (J.H. Kersey, personal communication). This registry is a most important first step, but still the main problem that remains is to determine if indeed, the tumor risk is increased in these patients, either as a total group or within individual disease categories.

The 2-10% risk for developing malignancies in the immunodeficient group (99) seems high, especially when compared
to a smaller group analyzed by Oleinik (93) or with the
analysis of the Registry's pediatric cases (100) in which
the only category which is clearly increased in the immunodeficient children as compared with normal children is the
lymphoreticular group including reticulum cell sarcoma,
lymphosarcoma, etc. The significance of the lymphoreticular
tumors can be questioned with the same arguments used for the
tumors appearing in immunodepressed organ transplant patients
concerning chronic antigenic stimulation and/or malignancies
of the target organs (88,89).

However, some interesting correlations can be seen in
patients with epithelial tumors. Such tumors are mainly
adenocarcinomas of the gastrointestinal tract and are associated with three main disease groups: ataxia-telangiectasia, common variable immune deficiency and IgA deficiency
(99). Based on the numbers and actual numbers of patients
at risk for these different categories obtained from the
Registry (99) it is difficult to ascertain if this correlation is valid, but some additional factors, such as age of
the patients (especially in the ataxia-telangiectasia group
in which ages ranged from 17 to 21 years, while the mean age
of the common variable immune deficiency group was approximately 50 years) are most suggestive (99).

A series of other diseases have been described in which
the incidence of malignancy is above average and in which no
detectable immune deficit has been detected. For example,
Fanconi's anemia is associated with a high incidence of
leukemia and squamous cell carcinomas(101,102). Klinefelter's
syndrome is associated with high incidence of leukemia and
lung carcinoma (103). (See reference 104 for a review of
these high-tumor-risk diseases). On the other hand, there
are some diseases which show both chromosomal abnormalities
as well as immune deficiencies and are associated with an
increase in tumor risk. Xeroderma pigmentosum has a high
incidence of skin tumors (105) and has deficiency of cell
mediated immunity (106). Similarly, patients with Down's
syndrome have a high incidence of leukemias and sarcomas
(107,108) but also show increased susceptibility to infections and depressed cell-mediated immunity (109). It should
be indicated that the fibroblasts of some of the patients
suffering from some of these diseases have an increased susceptibility to malignant transformation in vitro after exposure to SV40: this has been observed in Fanconi's anemia
(110), Klinefelter's (103) and Down's syndrome (110). On
the other hand, the fibroblasts of patients with the major

10

types of immunodeficiency disorders did not show such an increase in susceptibility to in vitro transformation by SV40 (111). However, the chromosomal defect may not be the sole factor in some of these situations; for example, the sibs of Down's syndrome patients have a high risk for leukemia development whether they have or do not have the syndrome (112,113). Similarly, the increased susceptibility to SV40 is not necessarily increased in all diseases associated with chromosome instability, since the fibroblasts of Xeroderma Pigmentosum patients do not transform more readily after exposure to the virus in vitro (114,115).

However, the alternative hypothesis used to deal with these cases was that there are two types of surveillance: one intrinsic to the cell (the chromosomal or other defects directly favoring the malignant changes) and another extrinsic to the cell (and most probably mediated by humoral and/or cell-mediated immunity) of which the immunodeficient patients would be the main example (116). Also, the predominance of lymphoreticular malignancies in the patients with primary immunodeficiency syndromes suggests that additional factors may also be of importance. Chronic antigenic stimulation of the lymphoid system, lack of immunoregulatory feedback mechanisms, infection or activation of endogenous oncogenic viruses, etc., may be operative (89,116).

In summary, there is suggestive evidence that immunosuppression, probably in association with other genetic and/or acquired defects, may be associated with a high incidence of primary malignancies. It is also apparent that a high incidence of primary malignancies can be associated with some genetic abnormalities in the absence of known immunological deficiencies (104). Thus, the case for "immune surveillance" at least in its orthodox presentation (55,56,58), seems not fully substantiated by the experimental and clinical data. Albeit, it has been and still is, one of the most provocative biological quandaries.

The last set of remarks concerns dogma and the rule-of-three (117). Immune surveillance has generated a large amount of research and a large amount of literature, especially in review form, and in many cases probably for brevity sake, some statements have been presented as absolute established facts. In "The Hunting of the Snark" the Bellman indicates that he has mentioned something three times and says: "What I tell you three times is true" (117). Thus, following this rule, statements repeated three times have a tendency to become established concepts. The association of malignancy with primary immunodeficiencies is a fascinating one, and a strong argument supporting the validity of immune surveillance. However, there are still several areas that deserve intensive study before the strength of such support is established.

REFERENCES

1. Good, R.A. (1973). Medicine 52: 405.
2. Gatti, R.A. and Good, R.A. (1970). Med. Clin. N. America 54: 281.
3. Bruton, O.C. (1952). Pediatrics 9: 722.
4. Gitlin, D. and Janeway, C.A. (1956). Progr. Hematol. 1: 318.
5. Page, A.R. and Good, R.A. (1960). J. Dis. Child. 99: 288.
6. Harington, H. (1828-1829).London Med. Gaz. 3: 314.
7. DiGeorge, A.M. (1968). In: Immunologic Deficiency Diseases in Man. Birth Defects Original Article Series Vol. 4, p. 116, National Foundation Press, New York.
8. Hitzig, W.H. and Willi, H. (1961). Schweiz. Med. Wschr. 91: 1625.
9. Gitlin, D. and Craig, J.M. (1963). Pediatrics 32: 517.
10. Hoyer, J.R., Cooper, M.D. et.al. (1968). Medicine 47: 201.
11. Fulginiti, V.A., Kempe, C.H., Hathaway, W.E. et.al.(1968). In: Immunologic Deficiency Diseases in Man. Birth Defects Original Article Series Vol. 4, p. 129, National Foundation Press, New York.
12. Matsaniotis, M. and Economou-Mavrou, C.(1968). In: Immunologic Deficiency Diseases in Man. Birth Defects Original Article Series Vol. 4, p. 124, National Foundation Press, New York.
13. Robbins, J.B. (1968). In: Immunologic Deficiency Diseases in Man. Birth Defects Original Article Series Vol. 4, p. 219, National Foundation Press, New York.
14. Murray, J.E., Wilson, R.E., Tilney, N.L. et.al.(1968). Ann. Surg. 168: 416.
15. Bach, M.C., Sahyoun, A., Adler, J.L. et.al. (1973). Transplant. Proc. 5: 549.
16. Barnes,B.A. et.al. (1972). 9th Report of the Human Renal Transplant Registry, JAMA 220: 253.
17. Ammann, A.J. and Hong, R. (1971). Medicine 50: 223.
18. Cooper, M.D., Chase, H.P.,Lowman, J.T. et.al. (1968). Amer. J. Med. 44: 499.
19. Baldini, M.G. (1969). New Eng. J. Med. 281: 107.
20. Peterson, R.D.A., Cooper, M.D. and Good, R.A. (1966). Amer. J. Med. 41: 342.

21. Seligmann, M., Fudenberg, H.H. and Good, R.A. (1968).
    Amer. J. Med. 45: 817.
22. Fudenberg, H.H. and Hirschhorn, K. (1965). Med. Clin. N.
    Amer. 49: 1533.
23. Good, R.A. (1973). In: The Harvey Lectures, Series 67,
    p. 1, Academic Press, New York.
24. Alper, C.A., Abramson, N., Johnston, R.B., Jr. et.al.
    (1970). New Eng. J. Med. 282: 349.
25. Day, N.K., Geiger, H., Stroud, R. et.al. (1972). J. Clin.
    Invest. 51: 1102.
26. Pickering, R.J., Michael, A.F., Jr., Herdman, R.C. et.al.
    (1970). J. Pediat. 78: 30.
27. Alper, C.A. and Rosen, F.S. (1971). Advan. Immunol. 14:
    251.
28. Berendes, H., Bridges, R.A. and Good, R.A. (1957). Minn.
    Med. 40: 309.
29. Holmes, B., Quie, P.G., Windhorst, D. and Good, R.A.
    (1966). Lancet I: 1225.
30. East, J.,Parrott, D.M.V., Chesterman, F.C. and Pomerance,
    A. (1963). J. Exp. Med. 118: 1069.
31. Stutman, O., Yunis, E.J. and Good, R.A. (1972). J. Exp.
    Med. 135: 339.
32. Mori, R., Takeya, K., Minamishima, Y. and Tasaki, T.
    (1965). Proc. Japan. Acad. of Sci. 41: 975.
33. Rees, R.J.W. (1966). Nature 211: 657.
34. Salvin, S.B., Peterson, R.D.A., and Good, R.A. (1965).
    J. Lab. Clin. Med. 65: 1004.
35. Preston, P.M., Carter, R.L., Leuchars, E. et.al. (1972).
    Clin. Expl. Immunol. 10: 337.
36. Schmunis, G.A., Gonzalez Cappa, S.M., Traversa, O.C. and
    Janovsky, J.F. (1971). Trans. Roy. Soc. Trop. Med. Hyg.
    65: 89.
37. Brown, I.N., Allison, A.C. and Taylor, R.B. (1968).
    Nature 219: 292.
38. Ogilvie, B.M. and Jones, V.E. (1967). Parasitology 57:335.
39. Domingo, E.O. and Warren, K.S. (1967). Am. J. Path.51:757.
40. Rowe, W.P., Black, P.H. and Levey, R.H. (1963). Proc.
    Soc. Exp. Biol. Med. 114: 248.
41. Flanagan, S.P. (1966). Genet. Res. 8: 295.
42. Pantelouris, E.M. (1968). Nature 217: 370.
43. Abelous, J.E. and Billard, A. (1896). Arch. de Physiol.
    Norm. et Path. 8: 898.
44. Ver Eecke, A. (1899). Bull.Acad.Roy. de Med. de Belg. 13:
    67.
45. Hammar, J.A. (1905). Arch.f.d.ges. Physiol. 110: 337.
46. Pari, G.A. (1905). Gazz.de.osp. (Bari) 26: 321.
47. Pari, G.A. (1906). Arch. Ital. de Biol. 46: 225.

48. Cooper, E.L. and Hildemann, W.H. (1965). Transplantation 3: 446.
49. Smith, C.H., Erlandson, M., Schulman, I. and Stern, G. (1957). Amer. J. Med. 22: 390.
50. Bogart, D., Biggar, W.D. and Good, R.A. (1972). J. Reticuloendothelial Soc. 11: 77.
51. Ehrlich, P. (1909). Nederlandsch Tijdscrift voor Geneeskunde 45:(la.) 273.
52. Thomas, L. (1959). In: Cellular and Humoral Aspects of Hypersensitive States, (Lawrence, H.S., ed.) p. 451, Hoeber-Harper, New York.
53. Brent, L. (1958). Progr. Allergy 5: 271.
54. Stutman, O. and Good, R.A. (1971). In: Advances in Biology of Skin. XI.Immunology and the Skin. (Montagna, W. and Billingham, R.E., eds.) p. 357, Appleton-Century-Crofts, New York.
55. Burnet, F.M. (1964). Brit. Med. Bull. 20: 154.
56. Burnet, F.M. (1970). Progr. Exp. Tumor. Res. 13: 1.
57. Good, R.A. and Finstad, J. (1969). Natl. Cancer. Inst. Monogr. 31: 41.
58. Good, R.A. (1972). Proc. Natl. Acad. Sci. USA. 69: 1026.
59. Penn, I. and Starzl, T.E. (1973). Transplant. Proc. 5:943.
60. Klein, G. (1973). Transplant. Proc. 5: 31.
61. Law, L.W. (1963). Nature 205: 672.
62. Ting, R.C. and Law, L.W. (1967). Progr. Exp. Tumor Res. 9: 165.
63. Kirschstein, R.L., Rabson, A.S. and Peters, E.A. (1964). Proc. Soc. Exp. Biol. Med. 117: 198.
64. Yohn, D.S., Funk, C.A., Kalnins, V.I. and Grace, J.T. (1965). J. Natl. Cancer Inst. 35: 617
65. Payne, L.N. (1972). In: Oncogenesis and Herpes Viruses; Proceedings of Symposium, p. 21, Cambridge University Press, New York.
66. Allison, A.C. and Law, L.W. (1968). Proc. Soc. Exp. Biol. Med. 127: 207.
67. Stutman, O. (1974). In: Proc. 1st Interntl. Workshop on Nude Mice (Rygaard, J. and Povlsen, C.O., eds.) p. 257, G. Fischer Verlag, Stuttgart.
68. Stutman, O. and Dupuy, J.M. (1972). J. Natl. Cancer Inst. 49: 1283.
69. Miller, J.F.A.P., Grant, G.A. and Roe, F.J.C. (1963). Nature 199: 920.
70. Grant, G.A. and Miller, J.F.A.P. (1965). Nature 205:1124.
71. Defendi, V. and Roosa, R.A. (1964) In: The Thymus. Wistar Institute Symposium Mon. #2. p. 121, Wistar Institute Press, Philadelphia.

72. Nomoto, K. and Takeya, K. (1969). J. Natl. Cancer Inst. 42: 445.
73. Law, L.W. (1966). Cancer Res. 26: 1121.
74. Balner, H. and Dersjant, H. (1966). J. Natl. Cancer Inst. 36: 513.
75. Allison, A.C. and Taylor, R.B. (1967). Cancer Res. 27:703.
76. Balner, H. and Dersjant, H. (1969). Nature 224: 376.
77. Cerilli, G.J. and Treat, R.C. (1969). Transplantation 8: 774.
78. Rabbat, A.G. and Jeejeebhoy, H.F. (1970). Transplantation 9: 164.
79. Fisher, J.C., Davis, R.C. and Mannick, J.A. (1970). Surgery 68: 150.
80. Wagner, J.L. and Haughton, G. (1971). J. Natl. Cancer Inst. 46: 1 .
81. Nehlsen, S.L. (1971). Clin. Exp. Immunol. 9: 63.
82. Stutman, O. (1972). Natl. Cancer Inst. Mon. #35: 107.
83. Stutman, O. (1974). Science 183: 534.
84. Trainin, N., Linker-Israeli, M., Small, M. and Boiato-Chen, L. (1967). Intl. J. Cancer 2:326.
85. Custer, R.P., Outzen, H.C., Eaton, G.J. and Prehn, R.T. (1973). J. Natl. Cancer Inst. 51: 707.
86. Rygaard, J. (1974). In: Proc. 1st Intl.Workshop on Nude Mice. (Rygaard, J. and Povlsen, eds.) p. 293, G.Fischer Verlag, Stuttgart.
87. Starzl, T.E., Penn, I., Putnam, C.W. et.al. (1971). Transplant. Rev. 7: 112.
88. Prehn, R.T. (1970). In: Immune Surveillance (Smith, R.T. and Landy, M., eds.) p. 451, Academic Press, New York
89. Schwartz, R.S. (1972). Lancet I: 1266.
90. Walder, B.K., Robertson, M.R. and Jeremy, D. (1971). Lancet II: 1282.
91. Metcalf, D. (1961). Brit. J. Cancer 15: 769.
92. Krueger, G.R., Malmgren, R.A. and Berard, C.E. (1971). Transplantation 11: 138.
93. Oleinick, A. (1969). J. Natl. Cancer Inst. 43: 775.
94. Oleinick, A. (1967). Blood 29: 144.
95. Moertel, C.G. and Hagedorn, A.B. (1957). Blood 12: 788.
96. Fraumeni, J.F., Jr., Manning, M.D. and Stark, C.R.(1964). JAMA 188:459
97. Gatti, R.A. and Good, R.A. (1971). Cancer 28: 89.
98. Waldmann, T.A., Strober, W. and Blaese, R.M. (1972). Ann. Inter. Med. 77: 605.
99. Kersey, J.H., Spector, B.D., and Good, R.A. (1973). Intl. J. Cancer 12: 333.
100. Kersey, J.H., Spector, B.D. and Good, R.A. (1974). J. Pediat. 84: 263.

101. Garriga, S. and Crosby, W.H. (1959). Blood 14: 1008.
102. Swift, M.R. and Hirschhorn, K. (1966). Ann. Inter. Med. 65: 496.
103. Mukerjee, D., Bowen, J. and Anderson, D. (1969). Cancer Res. 30: 1769.
104. Kundson, A.G., Jr. (1973). Adv. Cancer Res. 17: 317.
105. Cleaver, J.E. (1969). Proc. Natl. Acad. Sci. USA 63: 428.
106. Dupuy, J.M. and Lafforet, D. (1974). Clin. Immunol. and Immunopathol. 3: 52.
107. Krivit, W. and Good, R.A. (1956). Amer. J. Dis. Child. 91: 218.
108. McCormick, D.P., Meyer, W.J. and Nesbit, M.E. (1971). Amer. J. Dis. Child. 122: 71.
109. Sutnik, A.I., London, W.T., Blumberg, B.S. and Gerstley, B.J.S. (1971). US Natl. J. Cancer 47: 923.
110. Todaro, G.J., Grenn, H. and Swift, M.R. (1966). Science 153: 1252.
111. Kersey, J.H., Gatti, R.A., Good, R.A., Aaronson, S.A. and Todaro, G.J. (1972). Proc. Natl. Acad. Sci. USA 69: 980.
112. Miller, R.W. (1963). N. Eng. J. Med. 268: 393.
113. Miller, R.W. (1970). Ann. N.Y. Acad. Sci. 171: 637.
114. Aaronson, S.A. and Lytle, C.D. (1970). Nature 228: 359.
115. Parrington, J.M., Delhanty, J.D.A. and Baden, H.P. (1971). Ann. Hum. Genet. 35: 149.
116. Kersey, J.H. and Good, R.A. (1972). In: Membranes and Viruses in Immunopathology (Day, S. and Good, R.A. eds.) p. 277. Academic Press, New York.
117. Carrol, L. (1941). The Hunting of the Snark. p. 2. Chatto and Windus, London.

2

Immunosuppression by Murine Leukemia Viruses

Herman Friedman

INTRODUCTION

Although the nature and mechanism of virus-induced patho-
genicity has been the subject of countless investigations for
more than half a century, the effects of tumor virus infection and tumorigenesis on the host's immune responses has
only begun to be studied (6-10,14,18-21). This is ironic
since for over 80 years it has been well known that certain
virus infections can abrogate pre-existing cell-mediated immune responses. Diseases caused by viruses in both man and
experimental animals are often characterized by impairment of
normal lymphocyte functions, including antibody formation and
cellular immunity. The mechanisms by which a virus affects
the immune system, however, are still largely unknown.

The malignant transformation of normal cells by tumor viruses, both in vivo and in vitro is the subject of much current interest (6,13,19,20,22,24), but how the immune defense
mechanism influences such virus-induced tumors is, however,
largely uncharted. Many oncologists and immunologists believe that a functioning immune defense system is necessary
to prevent the emergence and proliferation of malignant cells
in vivo after virus-induced transformation (1,2,7,12,25).
Nevertheless, the manner in which virus-transformed tumor

cells "escape" from immune destruction is not understood.

One would expect that tumor-virus associated or induced antigens should stimulate an effective antitumor immunity since these antigens are presumably foreign even to the autochthonous host (16,25). Why, then, does the immune response mechanism fail to eliminate the virus-induced tumor? Several answers suggest themselves: a) The antitumor immune response of an individual may be too inefficient to deal with rapidly proliferating neoplastic cells after virus transformation; b) A tumor virus-associated-antigen(s) may be too "weak" to evoke a significant response. This could happen if an antigen were identical to, or cross reacted with, fetal antigens to which an individual would naturally be tolerant; c) Specific antitumor immunity, especially cell-mediated immunity, may be blocked by antibody, antigen-antibody complexes, or excessive antigen. This would prevent stimulation and/or activation of immunocompetent lymphocytes and the subsequent destruction of the transformed cells; d) A tumor virus per se may be immunosuppressive and actively interfere with the normal immunologic function of the infected host.

The last possibility has recently been studied in some detail to test the premise that tumors may be induced initially by a specific virus. In this regard, experimental models using various tumor viruses (especially those which induce lymphoreticular cell neoplasias) have shown that a generalized state of immunosuppression often accompanied virus-induced malignancy (6,8,10,19,20,22). Tumor viruses could impair immune responsiveness through a number of mechanisms. Among these is the possibility that, similar to some non-tumor viruses, the tumor virus directly damages or interferes with the function of such immune system cells as the T and B lymphocytes or macrophages (5,17,23,26). Alternatively, if a tumor virus induces a new antigen on normal lymphoid cells, such cells would then be recognized as "foreign" and stimulate an anti-lymphoid cell immunity directed to the virus-associated antigen(s) on the lymphoid cell per se. Such a response would be followed by destruction or injury of the lymphoid cells involved. Similarly, a localized or systemic antibody mediated (B cell) hypersensitivity reaction, rather than a T cell-mediated reaction, could be induced to the tumor virus antigen resulting in damage to virus antigen-containing lymphoid cells.

But this is a speculation. No one has yet shown how any virus, oncogenic or not, impairs immune function. It is known that some tumor viruses suppress immunologic capacity, some leave the immune functions unaffected, and others stimulate immune responses. Furthermore, those viruses which have demonstrable immunosuppressive properties may affect humoral immunity without influencing cell-mediated immunity, depress cell-mediated immunity without affecting humoral immunity, or suppress both forms of immunity.

Over the last eight years this laboratory has studied the immunosuppressive properties of murine RNA leukemia viruses using a research program illustrated in the schema (Fig. 1).

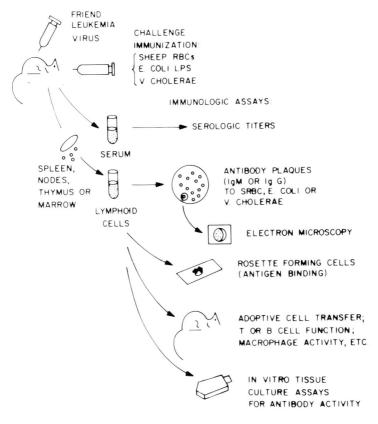

Fig. 1. Schematic representation of experimental model systems used to assess the interaction between murine leukemia viruses with various cells and pathways of the immune response to sheep erythrocytes, E. coli LPS, or Vibrio cholerae somatic antigen using immunobiologic assays.

The virus used for these studies has been the Friend leukemia virus (FLV) complex, which markedly affects humoral immunity and moderately affects cell-mediated responses. The complex

consists of at least two distinct components, the lymphatic
leukemia virus (LLV) and the spleen focus-forming virus(SFFV).

EFFECT OF FLV INFECTION ON HUMORAL ANTIBODY FORMATION TO SHEEP RED BLOOD CELLS (RBC)

Mice infected with FLV have a reduced ability to form circulating hemagglutinin and hemolysin during both primary and
secondary immune response to sheep red blood cell injection
(3,4,10). BALB/c mice injected with FLV 12 days before exposure to challenge immunization with 4 X 10^8 sheep RBC showed
markedly depressed serum hemolysin titers (Table 1, last col.)

Table 1: Effect of FLV dose on cellular PFC and humoral antibody
response to sheep erythrocytes after primary immunization.

Virus dose[a]	Spleen wt. (mg)	PFC/spleen	PFC/10^6 spleen cells	Serum hemolysin titer
None (saline)	128*	57,000	375	1:128
FLV 10^0	1560	1,200	5	1:2
10^{-1}	1275	2,400	6	1:2
10^{-2}	976	4,800	19	1:2
10^{-3}	315	7,300	60	1:16
10^{-4}	280	19,500	130	1:96

a
Balb/c mice injected i.p. with indicated dose of FLV 12 days before
challenge immunization with 4 x 10^8 sheep RBC ; all mice tested for
splenic 19S IgM PFCs and serum titers 4 days later.

and the larger the dose of FLV the greater the immunosuppression. The dose of RBC antigen used for challenge immunization also affected the level of immunosuppression since it
was possible to immunosuppress mice more effectively with
lower concentrations of FLV against 4 X 10^7 RBC than against
4 X 10^8 RBC.

Maximum immunosuppression occurred in mice infected with
FLV before RBC immunization. Infection of mice with FLV
8-13 days before RBC immunization resulted in a 5-10-fold or
greater depression in the peak hemagglutinin or hemolysin
titers. Infection 14-21 days before immunization resulted in
even greater suppression.

In contrast, mice given virus on the same day as RBC

immunization showed only moderate or no detectable suppression of serum antibody, while mice injected with virus even 1 or 3 days before immunization still showed significant immunosuppression. Mice infected with FLV <u>after</u> antigen challenge showed no suppression of response. Depression of serum antibody titers in infected mice was evident throughout the time of expected serum hemagglutinin or hemolysin formation, not only on the peak days of the response which generally occurred 7 to 10 days after challenge immunization. It seemed clear, therefore, that the degree of immunosuppression induced by FLV infection was related to the time interval between virus infection and challenge immunization and between the dose of virus and the dose of the antigen.

DEPRESSED APPEARANCE OF ANTIBODY FORMING CELLS IN INFECTED MICE

The availability of the hemolytic plaque assay for enumerating individual antibody plaque forming cells (APFC) permitted better quantitation of antibody responses (3,4,6,10, 11,20,22) to RBC following infection with FLV. For this purpose mice were infected with graded doses of virus and then challenged with sheep RBC exactly as for the serum antibody studies (Table 1, Figure 2). At various times after challenge immunization, representative control and infected mice were killed, their spleen and lymph node tissues excised aseptically and dispersed cell suspensions prepared. The number of APFCs against sheep RBC per spleen, per lymph node and per million lymphoid cells tested, was then determined by plaque assay in agar gel. A marked depression of APFCs similar to the results obtained at the serum hemolysin levels, occurred in the spleens of mice infected with FLV. The fewest APFCs appeared in spleens of mice infected for the longest time interval before challenge immunization as well as in those mice given the highest doses of virus (Table 1, Figure 2). Although greater immunodepression of the APFC response occurred later in the infection, a reduction in the expected number of APFCs was evident even in the spleens of mice given virus only one day before immunization. A 20-30% or even greater reduction occurred in mice infected for such a short time interval. However, mice infected with FLV 3-7 days or longer before challenge immunization showed much greater suppression, often with fewer than 5% to 10% of the number of splenic APFCs found in control mice. Enumeration of APFCs per million spleen cells tested showed an even greater depression, since splenomegaly was first observed at the end of the

21

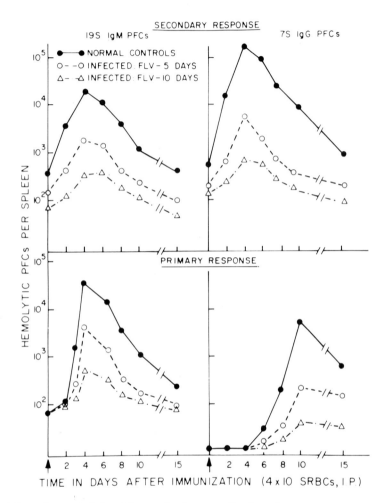

Fig. 2. Cytokinetics of the antibody plaque response to sheep erythrocytes in normal control and FLV-infected mice after primary and secondary immunization with RBC. Each point represents the average APFC response, either 19S IgM or 7S IgG, for 5 to 6 mice at the time indicated after challenge immunization. Secondary response determined in mice primed with same dose of sheep erythrocytes 4 to 5 weeks earlier. Infected mice injected IP with 10^{-1} dose FLV either 5 or 10 days before challenge immunization.

first week after infection. Mice challenged with antigen on
the same day as infection with FLV also showed a moderate
APFC suppression, especially on the peak or 4th day after immunization, or later. In contrast, mice given virus two days
after the sheep RBC, did not show any evidence of immunosuppression and, on occasion, actually had more APFCs on the
peak day after immunization (2 days after virus infection and
4 days after RBC injection).

Despite the marked differences in the magnitude of the
APFC responses in control versus infected mice, there was no
significant difference in the kinetics of the immune response
in infected animals when compared to controls, at least in
those mice challenged during the first 7-10 days after infection (when the leukemic process was first becoming evident
but APFC depression was still considerable) (Figure 2).
Markedly fewer APFCs were present on all assay days for infected versus control mice, regardless of the day of the response. For example, on day 2 after immunization, when the
rise in the number of APFCs began in normal mice, there was
a marked inhibition in infected animals. Similarly on day 3,
at the time of most rapid appearance of APFCs, there was
still a marked inhibition of APFC formation in infected mice.
After the peak day, when the number of APFCs declined rapidly
in the spleens of control mice, the number declined even more
rapidly in infected mice with the greatest decrease in those
mice infected for the longest time period and/or the highest
dose of viruses.

Depression of immunologic responsiveness at the cell level
was more evident for splenic APFCs of infected mice than for
lymph node APFCs. However, the ratio of splenic APFCs to
total lymph node APFCs was usually at least 20:1 in uninfected
mice. There was very little depression in the total number
of lymph nodes APFCs in infected mice during the first 7-14
days after infection when APFC responsiveness was markedly
diminished in the spleen of leukemic mice. Thus there was a
marked change in the ratio of splenic versus lymph node APFCs
in infected mice as compared to controls. This was due, however, to the depressed appearance of APFCs in spleens of infected mice and not to any significant change in the low numbers of lymph node APFCs in infected mice.

EFFECT OF INFECTION ON SECONDARY IgG ANTIBODY FORMING CELLS

The direct plaque assay used for enumerating APFCs in mice
immunized with sheep RBC mainly detected 19S IgM APFCs. However, late in the primary response and all during the secondary response to sheep RBC, low efficiency 7S IgG APFCs appeared. These were enumerated by an indirect hemolytic

facilitation assay using antiglobulin serum for enhancing IgG APFCs. The appearance of such low-efficiency APFCs in the spleen of mice given a single injection of sheep RBC after virus infection was significantly reduced as compared to non-infected control mice. Whereas peak numbers of IgG APFCs occurred on days 7 to 10 in both control and infected mice, their number in infected animals was generally 5-10-fold less than that observed in non-infected animals (Figure 2). The number of IgG APFCs appearing after secondary immunization with sheep RBC was even more suppressed in FLV-infected animals than the number of IgM APFCs.

Normal mice primed with sheep RBC 4 weeks before a second injection with the same dose of antigen have a rapid appearance of IgM and IgG APFCs, with the peak response 3-4 days after the booster immunization. In general, the number of IgG APFCs that appeared in the spleens of infected mice after booster immunization was fewer than that of IgM APFCs (Figure 2). The mice infected 7 days or longer before the booster injection showed the greatest degree of suppression (Figure 2). The level of immunosuppression during the secondary response was similar to that of the primary response and was directly influenced by the time interval between virus infection and booster immunization, as well as by the dose of virus. Maximum suppression occurred in mice given virus 7-14 days before secondary immunization. Animals given a 10^{-1} or 10^{-2} dose of virus showed a much greater depression of the IgG APFC response as compared to mice given lower doses of virus. The results of these experiments indicate that the "switch" of IgM to IgG hemolytic APFCs in RBC-immunized mice is rapidly suppressed in FLV-infected animals. This impairment is more pronounced than the depression of individual APFCs per se.

The nature and mechanism of this inhibition is unknown. However, the relatively greater suppression in the number of IgG APFCs in primed mice infected with FLV suggests that there may be an inhibition of "conversion" of IgM APFCs to the low efficiency hemolysin forming cells. This supports the belief that a similar cell line develops first into IgM and then into IgG antibody secreting cells.

ABSENCE OF A DIRECT AFFECT OF FLV ON MATURE ANTIBODY FORMING CELLS

The results of the APFC kinetic studies in mice infected with FLV were similar to those of other laboratories and support the concept that leukemia virus infection impairs immune responsiveness at the level of a "common" antibody precursor

cell, rather than in APFC per se. If FLV infection could
directly affect antibody synthesis at the level of individual
antibody forming cells per se, then one could expect that infection with virus after immunization would also depress
antibody competence. However, immunosuppression is most evident in mice infected prior to immunization. At that time,
antibody precursor cells are undoubtedly present and have not
yet been stimulated by antigen. The temporal relationship
suggests that virus infection might affect antibody formation
by "antigenic" competition, or more likely by a direct action
on "stem cells" and/or antibody precursor cells.

Before undertaking further studies to determine if these
explanations could account for the observed immunosuppression
in infected mice, it was necessary to determine if antibody
forming cells could be inhibited directly by FLV. For this
purpose, spleen cells from mice actively immunized with
sheep RBC were exposed to FLV in vivo and in vitro. In the
in vivo experiments, hemolysin-forming cells from immunized
control mice were transfered to non-immunized or X-irradiated
mice, which were then infected with FLV. No suppression of
the adoptively transferred APFCs could be detected regardless
of virus dose or time of FLV injection. In some cases there
was actually a slight enhancement of the adoptively transferred APFCs in recipients infected with FLV. Thus no direct
suppression of APFC function (i.e., antibody secretion) was
found in mice given transferred antibody-forming cells and
virus.

In an additional series of experiments, spleen cells from
RBC-immunized donors were transferred to FLV-infected mice.
The controls were normal or X-irradiated recipients. The
transferred APFCs persisted equally well in both (Table 2).
No diminution in the number of APFCs was noted in spleens of
mice given FLV before or after transfer of APFCs from RBC-
immunized donors. However, it should be noted that the
"homing" of APFCs into the spleen of infected versus control
mice might not be the same, since it has been reported that
the migration in vivo of lymphocytes in virus-infected mice
is impaired. Thus the detection of essentially the same number of transferred APFCs in the spleens of both infected and
control animals seems even more significant.

Studies in vitro confirmed these findings. Spleen cells
from sheep RBC-immunized-control mice were cultured in vitro
in the presence or absence of FLV either as an homogenate or
whole cell suspension from infected spleens. Earlier studies
had shown that spleen cells from FLV-infected mice challenged
in vivo with sheep RBCs do not form normal numbers of APFCs
upon subsequent culture in vitro. The marked in vivo suppres-

Table 2: Persistance of adoptively transferred hemolytic PFCs in
the spleens of normal and FLV infected recipients.

Day after spleen cell transfer[a]	PFCs transferred to recipient spleen[b]			
	Normal	FLV infected		
		+3 days	+8 days	+15 days
+1	346	295	430	315
+3	1165	1260	975	1130
+6	683	735	740	569
+10	173	215	198	165

a
Groups of normal or FLV infected (10^{-1} dose) Balb/c mice given 5×10^7
pooled spleen cells from syngeneic donor mice immunized 3-4 days earlier
with 4×10^8 sheep RBC .

b
Average number of splenic PFCs in 3-6 recipient mice on day indicated
after cell transfer.

sion continued under in vitro conditions, indicating that the
impaired response to sheep RBC was not due to a reversible
defect on the immunocompetent cells. In other experiments
spleen cells from non-infected normal mice were cultured.
The addition of sheep RBC to the cultures induced a marked
primary response, with large numbers of APFCs appearing 3-5
days later. Addition of FLV homogenates (cell-free extracts
of 7-10 day infected spleens) to the normal spleen cell cultures in vitro did not affect the expected APFC response.
On the other hand, when intact spleen cells from FLV-infected
mice were added to the normal spleen cells on the day of culture, there was a marked inhibition of the expected APFC response to the test erythrocytes (Table 3). Immunization in
vitro with sheep RBC did not stimulate a significant APFC
response in chambers containing either infected spleen cells
alone or chambers containing both normal and infected spleen
cells at a 10:1 ratio. Furthermore, even when infected
spleen cells were added one day after immunization in vitro
there was still a marked diminution of the expected APFC response. This in vitro impairment of immunity was dose-de-
pendent, in that the largest number of infected spleen cells
resulted in the lowest number of APFCs.
    Since cell-free FLV-containing extracts did not suppress
APFC formation in vitro, we asked whether virus associated

Table 3: Depressive ef'ect of FLV-infected spleen cells on in vitro immunization of normal mouse spleen cells.

Time in days of in vitro culture[a]	No additions	Infected spleen cells[b]	FLV homogenate[c]
0	5	4	5
+2	110	60	120
+3	320	110	310
+4	640	240	580
+5	975	310	870
+8	520	110	590
+10	240	60	310

a
  PFC for 3-5 in vitro cultures on day indicated after in vitro immunization of 5×10^6 spleen cells with sheep RBC .

b
  5×10^5 spleen cells from 10-15 day FLV injected mice added to spleen
  cultures at time of culture initiation and immunization.

c
  0.2 ml of 10% saline extract of infected spleen cells added to individual cultures at time of culture initiation and immunization.

with the leukemic cells was involved in the suppression in
vitro of normal APFC responsivenes. Infected cells were
separated from the normal spleen cells by Millipore membranes
in additional sets of culture chambers. Sheep RBC were added to the chamber containing normal spleen cells to be immunized. Infected cells, in graded numbers, were added to
the outer chamber. Under these conditions marked suppression
of APFC formation still occurred. The suppression, however,
appeared to be due to the FLV per se, since the addition of
mouse anti-FLV serum, with demonstrable neutralizing activity
for the virus, abolished the immunosuppressive property of
the leukemic cells. For example, when FLV serum was added to
either the leukemic cells in the outer chamber or to the target cells in the inner chamber no APFC suppression occurred.
These results indicate that infectious virus shed or budded
directly from leukemic cells either in direct contact with
normal spleen cells or when separated by Millipore membranes
could prevent the induction of an immune response in vitro
to sheep RBC. However, the same virus, when in a cell-free
homogenate, had no depressive effect on either induction of
APFCs or on antibody formation in vitro by spleen cells from
pre-immunized donors.

ULTRASTRUCTURE OF IMMUNOCYTES IN INFECTED MICE

The experiments described above support the earlier conclusions that antibody precursor cells were probably the
major site of virus-lymphoid cell interaction and that antibody forming cells per se were not directly affected by the
virus infection. This interpretation suggests a competition
exists between a leukemogenic virus and an antigen such as
sheep RBC for a "common" stem cell which, if first exposed to
antigen, develops into an antibody-forming cell. Virus infection, on the other hand, would divert the stem cell into
the pathway of leukemogenesis, rather than immunogenesis.
Those few antibody forming cells present in the spleen of
leukemic mice presumably would be the progeny of precursor
cells that had accidentally "escaped" infection at an earlier
stage.

Electron microscopic studies were therefore performed to
determine whether APFCs in the spleen of FLV-infected mice
were indeed free of evidence of infection. Control and infected mice were immunized with sheep RBC and plaque assays
performed. APFCs were selected and processed for electron
microscopy. Most hemolytic plaque cells from both control
and infected animals were of the lymphocytic series and appeared to be immature plasmablasts or immunoblasts. All anti-
body-producing cells examined from normal animals had highly
developed endoplasmic reticula and showed no evidence of
typical "C" type virus particles. The APFCs obtained from
the spleens of infected mice, although fewer in number, also
were typical lymphocytic cells and had highly developed endoplasmic reticula. Unexpectedly, a majority of these cells
contained type "C" particles, many of which were budding from
the cell membrane (Table 4). Over 55% of the APFCs from the
leukemic mice produced virus and synthesized hemolysins simultaneously.

These results indicated that antibody formation to sheep
RBC and infection with a leukemia virus of an individual
immunocyte is not a mutually exclusive event. It seems un-
likely, therefore, that immunologic impairment is due exclu-
sively to deviation of antibody precursor cells from the
pathway of immunogenesis to leukemogenesis. If this interpretation is correct, then no virus should have been present
in immunocytes producing antibody to the sheep RBC. However,
these results do not rule out the possibility that FLV infects precursor cells, deviating them from normal immune
function, since other cells after antigen stimulation might
have been infected at a later stage and continued to function
as antibody secreting cells for some time. Related studies

Table 4: Simultaneous presence of FLV virus particles and antibody
          formation in PFCs from infected mice.

Mouse group tested[a]	Number of PFC with "C" virus particles[b]
Normal	0/25
FLV infected −4 days	11/22
−8 days	13/20

[a]
PFCs examined from spleens of mice 4 days after challenge immuniza-
tion of normal or virus infected (10^{-1} dose) mice with 4×10^8 sheep
RBC .

[b]
Number of individual PFCs with typical "C" type virus particles
budding from cell membrane per number of PFCs examined by electron
microscopy.

with other viruses and immunologic systems also revealed that
leukemic cells may continue to form immunoglobulins and even
hemoglobulin at the same time that they show evidence of
active virus replication.

FLV EFFECTS ON ANTIGEN REACTIVE AND/OR ANTIBODY PRECURSOR CELLS

Although the ultrastructure studies indicated that leukemia virus infection and antibody formation were not mutually
exclusive, additional studies were performed to determine
whether antibody precursor cells were altered, either numer-
ically or functionally, in the spleens of FLV-infected mice.
For this purpose spleen cells from non-immunized FLV-infected
mice (i.e., not challenged with sheep RBC) were transferred
intravenously into X-irradiated mice, which were then challenged with the RBC. By this means it was possible to determine semi-quantitatively the number of "antigen reactive"
antibody precursor cells in the spleens of donor mice. This
was accomplished by counting both individual hemolytic foci
in intact sections of recipient spleens and individual APFCs
in dispersed recipient spleen cell suspensions. Each hemo-

lytic focus was considered to be the result of stimulation
of an antigen reactive precursor cell present in the donor
spleen cell population. Proliferation of these cells after
antigen stimulation would result in a cluster of APFC progeny
detectable as a hemolytic focus. Using this assay, it was
evident that the number of antigen reactive cells in the
spleens of FLV-infected mice decreased sharply. Within 3-5
days after FLV infection there were at least 50 to 60% fewer
precursor cells to the RBC antigens in FLV-infected mouse
spleen cells compared to the number present in control mice.
As the disease progressed, the number of cells capable of
reacting to sheep RBC after transfer to irradiated recipient
mice diminished even further.

The diminution in the number of such antigen-reactive cells
(foci-inducers), however, was not as great as that which
would be expected from the decreased number of APFCs in the
spleens of the same recipient. There was much greater depression in the number of APFCs versus hemolytic foci (Table 5).
Furthermore, the depressed focus and APFC response in the
recipients of spleen cells from FLV-infected donor mice was
not nearly as marked as the depressed APFC response which
occurred in similar leukemic mice challenged directly with
sheep RBC. Thus it appeared likely that together with the
marked depression in the number of antigen reactive cells in

Table 5: Decreased antibody precursor cells in spleens of FLV
infected mice assessed by adoptive transfer to irradiated mice.

Day after spleen cell transfer[a]	Spleen cells transferred[b]			
		FLV infected (days)		
	Normal	+3	+5	+10
+2	42	< 50	< 50	< 50
+4	85	< 50	< 50	< 50
+6	2065	125	120	113
+10	4735	768	341	142
+15	1150	175	98	81

a
Time in days after transfer of 5×10^7 spleen cells from indicated
donor group and challenge with sheep RBC .

b
Indicated spleen cells transferred i.v. to x-irradiated syngeneic mice;
average number of PFCs for 5-6 recipient mice on day indicated.

the spleens of infected animals there was also a defect in
the proliferative capacity of these cells. These results
point to a diminution in the number of detectable antigen-
reactive or antibody precursor cells in spleens of FLV-infected mice as at least a partial reason for immunodepression
during the course of Friend leukemia infection.

EFFECT OF FLV ON B AND T LYMPHOCYTES

It is now widely accepted that B and T lymphocytes must
collaborate synergistically in immunosuppressed recipient
mice to permit the appearance of hemolytic APFCs after challenge injection with sheep RBC. B lymphocytes alone are not
capable of providing the cell class necessary for immunologic
responsiveness to the response to RBC antigen. Although the
nature by which T cells collaborate with B cells is still
not known, we decided to see whether FLV-infection preferentially affected one or the other cell class, or both. Thymus
or bone marrow cells from either FLV-infected or normal control mice were injected intravenously, either together or
separately, into X-irradiated mice. These mice were then
challenged with sheep RBC and the number of individual APFCs
in their spleens was counted. Transfer of bone marrow and
thymus cells from normal donors to recipient mice readily
reconstituted immunity to sheep RBC. Transfer of either bone
marrow or thymus cells alone resulted in very few, if any,
APFCs. When thymus cells were derived from FLV-infected animals and marrow cells from normal donors, there was a normal
APFC response in the recipient mice (Figure 3). Similar
results were obtained with thymus cells from mice infected
with FLV for as short as 1 day or as long as 10-14 days. In
contrast, when bone marrow cells were transferred from FLV-
infected animals together with equivalent numbers of thymus
cells from normal donors into irradiated mice, there was a
markedly diminished APFC response after challenge immunization of the recipients (Figure 3). A 10-15-fold increase
in the number of marrow cells from FLV-infected donors did
not increase the response in the recipients. Thus, these
cell transfer studies indicated that B lymphocytes were the
most likely target of FLV-induced immunosuppression.
Additional studies with graded numbers of both thymus and
marrow cells from infected and control donors supported this
conclusion. However, in more recent experiments, some T
cells were affected, at least as far as helper-cell function
was concerned. Thymus cells obtained from mice infected 3
weeks or more with FLV showed significant impairment in their

31

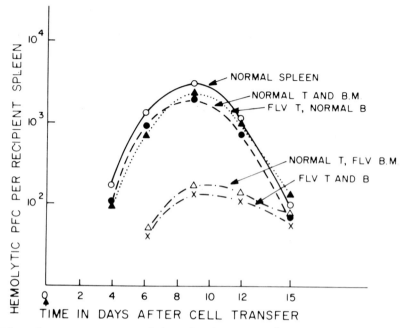

Fig. 3. Appearance of hemolytic APFCs in spleens of recipient mice X-irradiated 24 hours before challenge immunization (4 X 10^8 sheep RBC) and transfer of either spleen, thymus or bone marrow cells from normal or FLV-infected donor mice. Each point represents APFC response of 3 to 5 mice on day indicated after transfer of 5 X 10^7 cells to recipients and challenge immunization.

---

ability to collaborate with normal bone marrow cells in reconstituting immune responsiveness to sheep RBC. However, at this time the symptoms of leukemia were quite evident and most mice showed at least some evidence of severe disease.

ANTIGEN-BINDING ROSETTE CELLS IN FLV-INFECTED MICE

The cell transfer studies dealt mainly with functional capabilities and numbers of antigen reactive "stem cells" or antibody precursor cells in the B cell population of FLV-infected mice. The ability of this cell class to respond to sheep RBC was compromised in infected animals. However, only hemolytic antibody responses were measured.

It is now widely known that certain lymphocytes in all individuals can "recognize" sheep RBC and form clusters or

"rosettes" of RBC surrounding individual immunocytes. These
rosette-forming cells (RFC) are present in lymphoid tissues
of unimmunized mice and may represent antigen binding cells
with specific immunoglobulin receptors reactive toward RBC
antigens. Most of these RFC are thought to be T cells, although under some experimental situations, B lymphocytes from
unimmunized mice also form rosettes. After mice are immunized with sheep RBC the number of RFC increases markedly in
the spleen and lymph nodes. Most of these RFC represent B
lymphocytes reactive with the erythrocyte antigens, and some
may be the same cells recognized as APFCs by plating in agar
gel. This raises the question whether FLV infection affects
the number of RFC in spleen of mice before and after immunization with sheep RBC. To find out, mice were infected with
FLV at various times before challenge with RBC and were
studied for splenic RFC. Large numbers of "background" RFC
were present in the spleen and lymph nodes of control mice
before immunization. Such RFC were also present in the
spleens of FLV-infected animals, but their numbers were much
fewer, especially later in the course of infection (Table 6)
For the first few days after FLV injection the number of
"background" RFC decreased rather slowly. However, by days

Table 6: Rosette forming cells in spleens of normal and FLV infected
mice immunized with sheep RBC .

Time in days after challenge immunization[a]	Normal mice	Antibody RFC per spleen $(x10^3)$[b]				
				FLV infected		
		+1	+3	+7	+10	+15
0	7	6	1	<1	<1	<1
2	138	76	29	15	5	3
4	740	686	282	18	17	4
7	630	138	42	12	3	2
10	122	43	15	5	5	<1

a
Balb/c mice, either normal or FLV infected (10^{-1} dose), tested for
splenic RBC on day indicated before or after challenge injection
with 4 x 10^8 sheep RBC .

b
Average RFC response for 5-6 spleens for indicated mouse group.

7 to 10 there was a rapid decrease in their number, with even fewer present on days 20 to 25. A direct relationship was evident between both the dose and time of virus infection and the decrease in the number of RFC. Immunization of infected mice with sheep RBC resulted in decreased numbers of RFC (Table 6) relatively similar to the decrease in the number of APFCs. However, the relative decrease was not as great as that which occurred with APFCs. Nevertheless, by 7 to 10 days after infection with FLV, less than 5% of the normal number of RFC was present in the spleens of infected mice. This depression was only moderately less than that occurring at the level of APFCs. Thus the rosette assay for antigen binding cells indicated that even this parameter of immune competence was markedly impaired after FLV infection.

EFFECT OF FLV ON ANTIGEN PROCESSING AND PHAGOCYTIC CELLS

Over the last few years, many laboratories focused attention on the role of macrophages and/or other phagocytic cells in "antigen processing" during the initial stages of the immune response to sheep RBC. Odaka and others had indicated that FLV may infect macrophages directly (6,9). It seemed important, therefore, to determine whether phagocytic cell function in the immune response to RBC was affected by FLV infection. Earlier studies had revealed a dichotomous effect of FLV infection on phagocytic activity, i.e., early suppression followed by enhanced phagocytosis later in the course of the disease. To test for differences in antigen uptake, chromium 51-labeled RBC were injected intraperitoneally into both normal and FLV-infected mice. The uptake of the ^{51}chromium into the spleen and liver of the infected mice was then determined over a period of 24 to 48 hours. Essentially no difference was found between control and infected mice; however, 2-4 hours after RBC injection there was moderately less radioactivity in uninfected mouse spleens and livers, as compared to controls. Mice infected with FLV 2-10 days before testing all showed a slight to moderate decrease in RBC uptake during the first hours after challenge infection. However, by 24-48 hours there was no difference.

In corollary experiments, cell-free extracts from the tissues of mice at various times after RBC injection were injected into normal recipient animals. These were then tested for APFC formation 4-5 days later. A positive response was taken as evidence that an immunogen from the RBC persisted in the cell-free extract. There was essentially no difference in the persistence or localization of sheep RBC-immunogens between control and FLV-infected mice. The spleen and

liver extracts from infected mice had the same capacity to
stimulate a marked APFC response in "indicator" recipient
mice as did those from normal donor mice. Essentially equivalent values for RBC immunogen were obtained with FLV-infected and control mice. Therefore, impairment of phagocytic
activity of macrophages in mouse spleen or livers did not
account for the immunodepression evident in FLV-infected
mice.

EFFECT OF FLV ON IMMUNE RESPONSES TO BACTERIAL ANTIGENS -
DEPRESSED RESPONSE TO E. COLI SOMATIC ANTIGEN

Since the immune response to RBC antigens is not representative of all types of antibody responses, many studies
of the effects of tumor viruses on immunity have been based
on non-erythrocyte antigens (3,4,6,10,22). It is now widely
accepted that the immune response to several antigens, especially the lipopolysaccharide (LPS) somatic antigen of E.
coli, represents a "pure" B-cell immune response. Our laboratory, therefore, set out to determine whether infection of
mice with FLV would also suppress antibody formation to the
highly immunogenic E. coli LPS, as well as to somatic extracts from other Gram-negative bacteria. For these experiments, the direct bacteriolytic antibody plaque assay with
viable E. coli was used to assess the number of anti-coli
APFCs. When normal mice were injected with small doses of
E. coli LPS (5.0 to 50.0 μg), large numbers of bacteriolytic
APFCs appeared in their spleen within a few days, with peak
numbers on days 5-6. Mice first infected with FLV had considerably fewer bacteriolytic APFCs (Table 7). The rapid
decrease in the ability of the infected mice to form bacteriolytic APFCs, as well as serum agglutinins was similar to
the results with the sheep RBC system. Also, like the RBC
system, the time of infection and dose of virus markedly influenced the degree of immunosuppression.
To examine further the interaction of FLV on B lymphocyte
responsiveness, cell transfer experiments similar to those
with the sheep RBC system were performed with the E. coli
antigen. Both normal and FLV-infected donor mice were used
as the source of spleen, bone marrow, or thymus cells for
cell transfer. Transfer of spleen cells from normal versus
FLV-infected donors to X-irradiated recipients, followed by
challenge immunization with E. coli LPS, resulted in markedly
different responses. The spleen cells from normal donors
elicited large numbers of bacteriolytic APFCs in recipients;
spleen cells from the FLV-infected donors elicited very few

Table 7: Depressive effect of FLV infection on antibody response to E. coli in FLV infected mice.

Time in days after FLV injection[a]	PFC/spleen on day[b]					Serum agglutinin titer
	+3	+5	+8	+12	+15	
None (controls)	6,500	38,000	22,000	7,500	1,500	1:256
+2	7,000	41,000	28,000	6,900	1,800	1:256
0	6,100	18,500	11,500	3,400	1,100	1:128
-2	4,600	13,500	7,300	1,500	875	1:96
-5	2,500	11,300	5,000	1,100	‹50	1:32
-10	1,100	6,500	4,500	1,300	550	1:8
-15	750	3,500	2,100	950	350	1:8

a
 Groups of mice injected on day indicated, relative to day of infection, with 10^{-1} dose FLV.

b
 Average bacteriolytic PFC response of 5-6 mice on day indicated after immunization with E. coli LPS.

APFCs. Transfer of thymus cells from either donor group had little effect on the APFC response in the recipient mice, either when transferred alone or mixed with spleen or marrow cells from either group of donors. On the other hand, bone marrow cells from normal donors resulted in a significant APFC response to E. coli LPS in the recipients, indicating that these cells were capable of reconstituting the immune response to this antigen in irradiated recipients without the "help" of thymus cells. In contrast, bone marrow cells from mice infected with FLV 3-7 days or longer before testing were much less capable of reconstituting the immune response to E. coli LPS. Thus these results support the earlier conclusions that FLV infection affects B cell function preferentially since the adoptive transfer of immune responsiveness was inhibited not only to sheep RBC, a B cell antigen requiring the "help" of T cells, but also to E. coli LPS, an antigen considered T cell independent.

RESISTANCE OF A TRUE PRIMARY ANTI-VIBRIO IMMUNE RESPONSE TO FLV INFECTION

Earlier studies in this laboratory with Vibrio cholerae

36

somatic antigens indicated that the immune response to this antigen was due to B cell activation. However, a helper effect of T cells during the adoptive response to the vibrio antigens was consistently detected, although this effect was more pronounced for IgG than IgM responses. In the E. coli system only IgM APFCs were stimulated, with no IgG APFCs detected. On the other hand, mice injected with cholera somatic antigen formed large numbers of both IgM and IgG vibriolytic APFCs. These could be detected by plating spleen cells in agar gel containing living cholera bacilli. Late in the primary response and during the secondary response low efficiency vibriolytic APFCs were readily detected with antiglobulin serum by methods similar to those used for detecting low efficiency APFCs to RBC antigens. The immune response to the vibrio bacilli differed significantly from those to other antigens such as RBC or E. coli LPS. Mice respond with what appears to be a "true" primary response to vibrio. No "background" pre-existing antibody forming cells are present in the spleen or lymph nodes of normal mice before immunization with the cholera antigens. Furthermore, there is a delay of at least 42-44 hours before the first APFCs appear after immunization, followed by a slow increase in their number until the peak of the response, which occurs on days 12-14 after immunization, rather than at days 4-5 as with sheep RBC or E. coli antigen. Thus the absence of pre-existing APFCs to cholera bacilli and the marked delay before the peak of the APFC response indicate that mice respond to this antigen with a true primary response.

It was, therefore, of obvious interest to determine whether FLV infection affected the response to the vibrio antigens. Despite the known difference between immune responses to cholera bacilli vs. other antigens, it was still surprising to find that APFC formation to the cholera antigen was largely unaffected by FLV infection, at least early in the course of the disease. Mice given an inoculum of FLV known to rapidly depress the immune response to RBC or E. coli LPS showed no impairment of immunity to the vibrio antigen (Table 8). For example, infection of mice 1-3 days after challenge immunization with heat-killed vibrios did not suppress the expected vibriolytic APFC (Table 9). Indeed FLV-infected mice actually had enhanced antibody response,to the cholera bacilli. When FLV was given simultaneously with or after immunization with vibrios there was a consistent enhancement of the vibriolytic APFC response, especially on the peak days. These results, therefore, suggest that a "true primary" antibody response is resistant to FLV-induced immunosuppression. To test this possibility further,

37

Table 8: Peak vibriolytic PFC response in spleens of mice after primary
or secondary immunization with cholera vaccine and injection
with FLV.

Mouse group tested[a]	Vibriolytic PFCs per spleen[b]		
	Primary response (IgM)	Secondary response[c] IgM	IgG
Normal controls	59,500	65,000	18,500
FLV infected −0 day	73,100	31,000	20,000
−1 day	81,500	28,000	13,000
−3 days	62,100	10,000	11,000
−6 days	48,200	10,100	7,500
−9 days	31,600	6,300	3,000

a
Mice injected i.p. with 10^{-1} dose of FLV on indicated day relative to
day of challenge immunization with 50 µg V. cholerae vaccine.

b
Average response of 4-6 mice per group 12 days after primary immunization or 8 days after secondary immunization.

c
Mice primed i.p. with cholera vaccine 8 weeks before secondary immunization.

Table 9: Comparative suppression of primary and secondary PFC responses
to different test antigens in mice infected with FLV.

Test antigen[a]	Percent of control[b]		
	Primary response (IgM)	Secondary response (IgM)	(IgG)
Sheep erythrocytes (4 x 10^8 RBCs)	3.2	5.2	2.1
E. coli LPS (50 µg)	5.6	6.3	---
V. Cholerae vaccine (50 µg)	12.5	10.1	6.5

a
Mice injected with 10^{-1} dose of FLV 3-6 days before primary or secondary
challenge immunization with indicated antigens.

b
Average percent of control response at peak of expected primary or secondary responses of infected vs. non-infected control mice.

additional experiments were performed with mice first primed
with cholera bacilli and then infected with FLV followed by
a booster immunization with the same vibrio vaccine eight
weeks later. A marked secondary APFC response invariably
developed in control primed mice, characterized by the rapid
appearance of IgM and IgG APFCs (Table 9). In contrast, mice
infected with FLV several days before the booster immunization with vibrios showed a marked suppression of the expected
APFC response. This suppression was similar to that which
occurs when FLV-infected mice were immunized for the first
time with either sheep RBC or E. coli antigen. The main difference between primary and secondary immune responses to the
cholera antigen and other test antigens appeared to be the
presence or absence of vibriolytic APFCs at the time of FLV
infection. The absence of vibriolytic APFCs before primary
immunization and their presence before secondary immunization
may be an important factor in terms of the effect of FLV infection on the immune response. The leukemia virus-induced
immunosuppression appeared to be affected more by the nature
of the immune response involved rather than the antigen per
se. The true primary response, represented by the APFC response to a single injection of cholera vaccine, seemed unaffected by FLV infection, at least early in the course of the
disease. This has been interpreted as reflecting a greater
"preference" of the FLV for those cells or immunocytes that
have already been "activated" by antigen stimulation. Cells
not yet activated by antigen are less "mature" and in a
"quiescent" state. Perhaps they have lower metabolic activity and do not provide the biochemical apparatus needed for
virus replication.

GENETIC RESISTANCE TO FLV-INDUCED IMMUNOSUPPRESSION

Recent studies of FLV infection have shown that this leukemogenic virus exists as a complex: one component is the
lymphatic leukemia virus (LLV); the other is the spleen
focus-forming virus (SFFV). Both virus components seem necessary for maximum immunosuppression (6,11,20). Furthermore,
genetic loci control susceptibility to FLV infection. Genetic
studies of different strains of mice have revealed the existence of two major loci for resistance and immunosuppression
(FV-1 and FV-2, respectively). Certain strains of leukemia
virus-susceptible mice, such as BALB/c and DBA/2, have a
similar FV-2 genotype, designated s, but differ at the FV-1
locus, which controls susceptibility to the N-and B-tropic
strains of the LLV component of the FLV complex. Thus,

BALB/c mice have the genotype $FV-1_b$, $FV-2_s$ and DBA/2 mice
have the genotype $FV-1_n$, $FV-2_s$. These mouse strains are
highly susceptible to FLV-induced leukemia and show marked
depression of antibody responsiveness after challenge immunization with a variety of antigens, including sheep RBC and
E. coli LPS. Possession of the $FV-2_s$ genotype appears to
control both susceptibility to disease and to immunologic impairment. On the other hand, FLV-resistant mouse strains,
exemplified by C57Bl/6 mice, do not develop symptoms of leukemia when infected with FLV or its components. We asked
whether these resistant mice would show evidence of immunosuppression when challenged with sheep RBC.

Injection of FLV into C57Bl/6 mice 1,3,7 or 10 days before
challenge immunization with sheep RBC resulted in a dichotomous response. Normal mice of this strain responded with
large numbers of hemolytic APFCs with the peak 4-5 days after
immunization. FLV-infected mice showed both normal and impaired responses, depending upon the time between immunization and infection. Mice given FLV 1-3 days before challenge
immunization showed a markedly depressed APFC response; mice
injected with virus 7-10 days after immunization showed a
completely normal response (Table 10). Thus a significant

Table 10: Genetic control of susceptibility to FLV infection and immunosuppression demonstrable by challenge infection and immunization of different strains of mice.

Time in days between infection and immunization[a]	Balb/c		C57Bl/6	
	PFC/spleen	FLV present	PFC/spleen	FLV present
Controls (no FLV)	75,100	–	56,700	–
FLV infected -1 day	12,000	+	6,800	+
-3 days	3,750	+	2,300	+
-7 days	585	+	62,000	–
-10 days	260	+	61,000	–

a
Groups of mice injected with 10^{-1} dose of FLV on indicated day before challenge immunization with 4×10^8 sheep RBCs; average number of splenic PFC
and detectable FLV determined for both mouse strains 4 days later.

although temporary immunosuppression occurred in the C57Bl/6
mice injected with FLV shortly before challenge immunization.
Similar results were observed for the secondary response to
sheep RBC. It is noteworthy that none of the FLV-infected
C57Bl/6 mice showed evidence of leukemia. However, cell-free
extracts from the spleen or other lymphoid organs of these
mice obtained during the first 5-8 days after infection induced marked splenomegaly when injected into BALB/c

and C57Bl/6 mice. No infectious virus was detected 10 days or more after FLV injection into the C57Bl/6 mice. Thus the temporary immunosuppression in the C57Bl/6 mice seemed related directly to the persistence of FLV in these "resistant" mice. Virus replicated in these mice and titration by either in vitro or in vivo assays showed increasing numbers for a period of 5-6 days after infection, and then a rapid decrease.

MECHANISMS AND SIGNIFICANCE OF FLV-INDUCED IMMUNOSUPPRESSION

The primary goal of these studies from our laboratory was to assess the nature, mechanism and significance of the interaction of a tumor virus with cells of the immunologic response system. A leukemia virus can suppress immune responsiveness, especially antibody formation, by a number of modalities. For example, it may directly affect the function of immunocompetent cells thereby depressing antibody formation (Figure 4). An additional possibility is that a leukemia virus infects lymphoid cells but the infection is not

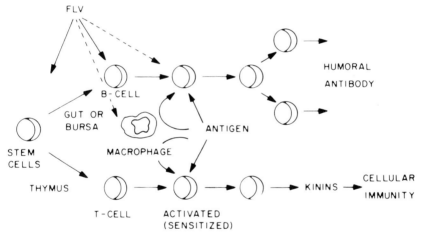

Fig. 4. Schematic representation of pathways of immune responsiveness to antigen stimulation by cellular (T-lymphocyte) and humoral (B-lymphocyte) immune systems. FLV may interact with different cell classes involved in the humoral immune response as indicated by solid and dashed arrows, especially with cells which are either stem or precursor cells for antibody formation.

lytic, i.e., the virus replicates without killing the lymphoid cells. However, such virus-infected cells would undoubt-

41

edly develop leukemia virus-associated surface antigens,
which, in turn, might stimulate an anti-lymphocyte response
by other cells. Immune responses to such tumor virus associated antigens may result in a local or systemic anti-tumor
immune response, culminating in either direct or indirect
destruction of the lymphoid cells. It is also possible that
tumor virus-induced immunosuppression is due to events unrelated to antibody formation per se. Excessive amounts of
tumor-antigen-antibody complexes could be immunosuppressive
by "blockading" phagocytic cells or other cells of the reticuloendothelial system (RES). Alternatively, serum antigen-
antibody complexes may result in formation or release of
pharmocologically active substances which are indirectly immunosuppressive.

The results of studies described above, as well as studies
from other laboratories, suggest that antibody precursor or
antigen-reactive stem cells are affected by leukemia virus
injection   (Figure 4). Inhibition or alteration of these
cells could affect the immune response mechanism, especially
if these cells were diverted from the pathway of antibody
formation into the pathway of leukemogenesis (6,10,11,22,24).
The current concept that tumor viruses interact with a common stem, which can be either stimulated by antigen to develop into an immunocompetent cell or alternatively, infected
by tumor viruses and transformed into a leukemic cell, is
presently in some dispute. For example, the finding that
leukemia virus particles "bud" from the surface of antibody-
synthesizing cells indicates that even immunocytes already
stimulated by antigen may be infected by virus. The complex
relationship between the immunocompetence of individual immunocytes and susceptibility or resistance to infection by a
leukemia virus is exemplified further by studies with vibrio
bacilli. As discussed before, it seems evident that a true
primary immune response to cholera antigens is largely unaffected by FLV infection early during the course of the disease.

Thus some immune responses may be resistant to FLV-induced
immunosuppression. This finding may have a much broader implication than the mere observation that an immune response
to a certain antigen is unaffected by a leukemogenic virus.
It seems significant that secondary but not true primary
immune responses may be more susceptible to virus induced immunosuppression. This may mean that antigen-activated cells
are the preferential cell type for leukemia virus replication.
Thus those cells previously stimulated by antigen either by
direct immunization or by inapparent exposure of the individual to the same or cross-reacting antigens in the environment

42

are more readily infected by tumor virus and can support a more rapid or efficient replication of the virus than non-activated lymphoid cells (10,15,27). There is evidence in the literature that cells stimulated by non-specific mitogens or other agents can support the replication of various viruses much better than unstimulated cells (15,27). Virus replication in an antibody-synthesizing cell or its precursor may result in the appearance of virus-associated antigen(s) on the surface of the immunocyte. Such an antigen could then stimulate an "autoimmune" response against the tumor-antigen-bearing lymphocytes. This could then result in the selective destruction of those cells that had been stimulated by an antigen and infected with the virus.

In the above postulated scenerio, cell destruction could be accomplished either by sensitized lymphoid cells, presumably T cells, or by anti-virus antibody and complement. Thus some evidence of anti-tumor immunity should be detectable in a leukemia virus-infected individual, at least early in the course of the disease before the entire immune mechanism becomes affected or before possible "excessive" tumor antigen would inhibit or block detection of a specific anti-tumor immunity.

It is also possible that a leukemogenic virus depresses the host genome increasing the level of embryonic antigens on the surface of an infected immunocyte. Such derepressed fetal antigens on the lymphocyte surface could act as an antigenic determinant similar to that of the tumor virus itself and stimulate an immune response. It seems noteworthy that other investigators, using different approaches, have come to similar conclusions that leukemogenesis may be associated with an "autoimmune" process (15,19). It has been postulated recently that when the host makes an inadequate immune response against tumor antigens, the tumor cells proliferate and kill the host; when host immunity is adequate, the tumor is eventually destroyed. Tumors induced by RNA viruses would elicit antinucleic acid immune responses. Thus autoimmune diseases characterized by antinucleic acid antibodies in the serum might be the result of a successful defense by the immune system against a tumor virus. Therefore, in some situations autoimmunity and leukemogenesis may be closely related. The greater susceptibility of antigen-stimulated lymphoid cells to tumor virus replication may be the major reason for an apparent selective destruction of immunocompetent B cells. If this view is correct, then it would seem likely that activated T cells capable of interacting with tumor virus antigens should be present during the course of virus leukemia. Other studies not described here have shown that FLV infec-

tion, although inducing a marked impairment of antibody formation, results in a less severe depression of cell-mediated
immunity to unrelated antigens, such as allografts or myco-
bacterial antigens, at least early in the course of the disease. However, after a moderate delay, a marked depression
of cell-mediated immunity does occur. A relatively "normal"
cellular immunity early in the course of Friend leukemia, if
it exists, may permit an "autoimmune" response mediated by
activated T cells, either against the virus-associated antigen per se or against the virus-transferred, antibody-pro-
ducing cell. Neutralizing antibody formed by B cells may be
protective against the virus. Inhibition of B cell responsiveness by the virus might protect the virus from immune
destruction. An effect on T cell immunity would provide the
final blow by inhibiting those very immunocytes which might
be protective against the virus-induced disease.

The possible mechanisms outlined above for generalized
tumor-virus-induced immunosuppression may also be the mechanism for the temporary immunodeficiency occurring in FLV-
resistant mouse strains. However, suppression appears to be
limited only to the B cell response in leukemia virus-resist-
ant mice, since cellular immunity is not affected, even temporarily. Similarly, non-oncogenic viruses often suppress
immune responses, at least temporarily. Therefore, the
ability of an infected individual to recover from a temporary
suppression may be basic to the eventual outcome of the virus-host interaction. Immune response genes related to both
histocompatibility genes and virus-susceptibility genes appear to have a direct bearing on the tumor virus interaction
with the host immune defense mechanism and the eventual development of a progressing neoplastic disease.

The depression of immunologic competence to both virus
antigens and virus-unrelated antigens during leukemia virus
infection may be a necessary prerequisite for the leukemogenic process. This possibility has been discussed above and
in detail by a number of other investigators (2,6,9). Experimental studies have not yet demonstrated that immunosuppression is an unequivocal requirement, especially since tumor
viruses can induce malignant transformation in vitro in the
absence of any functioning immune system. However, the eventual progression of transformed cells in vivo may depend on
the impairment, either direct or indirect, of the host's
defense mechanism to either respond to, or interact with, the
transformed malignant cell. There seems little doubt now
that a complex interrelationship exists between tumor virus
infection, the immune response mechanism, and the tumorigenic
process itself.

CONCLUSIONS AND SUMMARY

Recent studies have shown that murine RNA leukemogenic viruses are immunosuppressive. Deficiencies in a variety of antibody responses are consistently observed in leukemia virus-infected mice. The mechanism of such virus induced immunosuppression is, however, not fully understood. Immunosuppression may be due to direct effects of tumor virus infection on different cell types involved in various pathways of the immune response. Studies with the FLV model have permitted extensive analyses of various effects of leukemia virus infection on different parameters of antibody formation. Infection of mice with FLV suppresses the primary immune response to sheep RBC and E. coli LPS. Both 19S IgM and 7S IgG hemolysin-forming cells are markedly suppressed in FLV-infected mice challenged with sheep RBC, with greater depression of the 7S response than 19S response. The time interval between virus infection and challenge immunization, as well as the dose of virus, affected the response. Antigen reactive cells or antibody precursor cells in the B lymphocyte population were the main target for immunosuppression. The numbers of antigen-binding cells for sheep RBC, both in non-immune and RBC-immunized mice, were also markedly suppressed. In vitro studies indicated that virus-infected leukemic cells, but not cell-free virus, could prevent in vitro immunization of normal spleen cells. There was no inhibitory effect on antibody-forming cells directly. Electron microscopy showed the presence of typical leukemia virus particles budding from the surface of many lymphoid cells in the process of secreting antibody to RBC. Thus leukemia virus infection and antibody formation are not mutually exclusive events at the level of individual immunocompetent cells. FLV infection did not significantly affect the antigen processing mechanism and/or phagocytic cells.

A true primary immune response to vibrio cholerae somatic antigen was not affected by FLV infection. In contrast, the secondary immune response to vibrios was readily suppressed, suggesting that antigen-stimulated or antigen-activated immunocompetent cells may be more susceptible to virus infection. The sum total of these studies of the effects of FLV infection on antibody formation indicates that immunosuppression is due mainly to virus-induced alteration of antibody precursor cells per se, or alternatively, to the preferential infection of antigen-activated lymphoid cells, with a concomitant "autoimmune" response to those cells after they acquire leukemia virus-associated antigens on their surface.

The investigations in the author's laboratory were supported by research grants from the American Cancer Society (T138), and U.S. National Science Foundation (GB 6215X) and the National Institutes of Health (AI 10113).

Acknowledgements

Most of the experiments described from the author's laboratory were performed with the enthusiastic and excellent cooperation and collaboration of Dr. Walter S. Ceglowski, Pennsylvania State University. In addition, various phases of these studies were performed with the excellent collaboration of Drs. J. Allen, J. Cerny, S. Hirano, I. Kamo and J. Kateley, Jr. The excellent technical assistance of Mrs. Leony Mills, Miss Joyce Janderowski, Miss Marcia Israel and Miss Lois Fenner during various portions of these studies is also acknowledged.

REFERENCES

1. Burnet, F.M. (1969). Cellular Immunology, Cambridge Univ. Press, Australia.
2. Burnet, F.M. (1970). Immunological Surveillance. Pergamon Press, New York.
3. Ceglowski, W.S., LaBadie, G.U. and Friedman, H. (1973). Adv. in Exp. Med. & Biol. 29: 499.
4. Ceglowski, W.S., LaBadie, G.U.,Mills, L. and Friedman, H. (1973). In: Virus Tumorigenesis and Immunogenesis. (Ceglowski, W.S. and Friedman, H., eds.) p.167, Academic Press, New York.
5. Claman, H.N. and Chaperon, E.A. (1969). Transpl. Rev.1:92.
6. Dent, P.B. (1972). Progr. Med. Virol. 14:1.
7. Fairley, G.H. (1969). Brit. Med. Bull. ii: 467.
8. Friedman, H. (1974). Israel J. Med. Sci. 10:1052.
9. Friedman, H. and Ceglowski, W.S. (1971). Progr. Immunol. 1: 815.
10. Friedman, H. and Ceglowski, W.S. (1974). In: Role of Immunologic Factors in Viral and Oncogenic Processes. (Beers, R.F., Tilghmann, R.C. & Basset, E.G., eds.) p. 187, Johns Hopkins Univ. Press, Maryland.
11. Friedman, H. and Ceglowski, W.S. In: Proc. M.D. Anderson Symp. (Hersch, M.E. and Schlamowitz, M., eds.) In Press.
12. Good, R.A. and Finstad, J. (1968). In: Proc. Internatl. Conf. Leukemia-Lymphoma. (Zarafonetis, C.J.D., ed.) p. 175, Lea and Febiger, Philadelphia, Pa.

13. Gross, L. (1970). Oncogenic Viruses, 2nd ed. Pergamon Press, London.
14. Hellström, K.E. and Hellström, I. (1970). Ann. Rev. Microbiol. 24: 373.
15. Hirsch, M.S. (1974). In: Role of Immunologic Factors in Viral and Oncogenic Processes. (Beers, R.F., Tilghmann, R.C. and Basset, E.G., eds.), p. 177, Johns Hopkins University Press, Maryland.
16. Isacson, P. (1967). Progr. Allergy 10: 256.
17. Lerner, R.A. and Dixon, F.J. (1973). Scientific American 228: 82.
18. Liebowitz, S. and Schwartz, R.S. (1971). Adv. Int. Med. 17: 95.
19. Notkins, A.L. and Koprowski, H. (1973). Scientific American 228: 22.
20. Notkins, A.L., Mergenhagen, S.E. and Howard, R.J. (1970). Ann. Rev. Microbiol. 24: 525.
21. Penn, I. and Starzl, T.E. (1972). Transpl. 14: 407.
22. Salaman, M.H. (1969). Antibiotica et Chematherapia 15:393.
23. Schwartz, R.S., Ryder, R.J.W. and Gottlieb, A.A. (1970). Progr. Allergy 14: 81.
24. Siegel, B.V. and Morton, J.I. (1973). In: Virus Tumorigenesis and Immunogenesis. (Ceglowski, W.S. and Friedman, H., eds.), p.271, Academic Press, New York.
25. Sjögren, H.O. and Bansal, S.C. (1971). Progr. Immunol. 1: 921.
26. Talmage, D.W., Radovich, J. and Hemmingsen, H. (1970). Adv. Immunol. 12: 271.
27. Wheelock, E.F., Toy, S.T. and Stjernholm, R.I. (1971). Progr. Immunol. 1: 787.

3

Restoration of Immunologic Competence in Viral Leukemogenesis

E. Frederick Wheelock

IMMUNODERANGEMENTS

One of the most important objectives in cancer research today is determination of the role that the immune system plays in resistance against neoplastic disease. Supporting the importance of such a role is the high incidence of neo-plastic disease occurring in patients with congenital immune deficiency syndromes and in organ transplant recipients who receive intensive immunosuppressive therapy (1). In addition, many patients with malignant disease demonstrate an impair-ment in one or more components of their immune system (2). The central question is whether these impairments are causal, consequential, or incidental to the neoplastic process; that is, does the neoplasm develop because there is a defect in the patient's immune system resulting in diminished resist-ance to a new tumor antigen or does the neoplastic process itself involve immune cells and in this way produce immuno-suppression, or are the two disconnected.

Depression of both immune and non-immune host defense mechanisms in patients with a variety of malignancies is a frequent occurrence and has been used as a sign of poor prognosis (3,4,5). Attempts are currently being made to restore and stimulate immune and non-immune host responses to tumor cells in an effort to enhance host resistance to neoplastic disease. These efforts include both specific and non-specific, active and passive immunotherapy (6,7).

In support of a causal relationship between immunocompe-tence and response to chemotherapy is a study by Hersh et al. (5) who evaluated the immunocompetence of 25 patients with acute myologenous leukemia before and after intensive com-

bination chemotherapy for induction of remission. They found
that cell mediated immunity (CMI) correlated with response to
chemotherapy. Patients converting from immuno-incompetence
to immunocompetence during therapy achieved remission, whereas those converting from immunocompetence to immuno-incompetence did not. Harris et al.,(4), emphasized the importance
of the pattern of immune recovery after chemotherapy of malignant disease as the most valuable prognostic determinant
of clinical response. Lymphocyte reactivity was consistently
3 to 12 times higher in patients who responded clinically to
chemotherapy. These studies indicate the value of serial
multivarient immunologic evaluations in patients undergoing
cancer chemotherapy, and suggest a causal relationship between the degree of immunocompetence of the patient and a
clinical response to anti-tumor treatment. Central to these
studies is the importance of evaluating competence of the
specific host function that is directly involved in defense
against the tumor carried by the host.

In animal model systems, immunosuppressive drugs have been
shown to enhance the oncogenic effects of a number of viruses
(8), and increase the incidence of cancer in animals genetically predisposed to such cancers (9). Severe prolonged
immunodepression by itself, however, has failed to promote
the development of lymphomas in animals not predisposed to
such neoplasms(10). In contrast, no clear relationship has
been established between immunodepression and the development
of malignant disease following graft vs. host reactions (11).

The murine leukemia virus models are biological systems
which have been extensively employed by investigators inter-
ested in this problem. Infection of DBA/2 mice with Friend
virus (FV) produces immunodepression involving both humoral
and cellular immunity followed by a rapidly fatal erythroleukemia. Depression of the immune response to sheep erythrocytes (SRBC) in FV infected mice was first reported by Old
and his associates in 1960 (12). These observations have
been corroborated and extended by the investigators (13).
Wedderburn and Salaman (14) found that SRBC antigen uptake
by the spleen was not impaired during FV leukemogenesis.
Friedman and Ceglowski (15) (also see Chapter 3) conducted
cell transfer experiments with irradiated mice and concluded
that the FV induced reduction in SRBC antigen plaque forming
cell production lay in the "B" cell population in the form of
a proliferative defect. Similar conclusions were reached by
Salaman (16). Bennett and Steeves (17) also found a defect in
the precursors of antibody forming "B" cells and in addition,
presented evidence that "T" cell function remained intact.
Certain subpopulations of "T" cells however, probably do have

FV-induced defects as shown by the depressed PHA response found in cell populations of Rauscher virus infected mice(18), and depression of MIF activity in FV infected mice (19).

Evidence exists that depression of humoral immunity may be requisite for virus induced leukemias (20). In addition, strains of mice which are resistant to erythroleukemogenic viruses have been reported by some (21,22,23,24,25) but not all (26,27) investigators to be also resistant to the immuno-depressive effects of these viruses. However, immunodepression alone may not be sufficient for the establishment of the rapidly fatal acute leukemia seen in FV infections; the Rausson-Parr virus (LLV) isolated from the FV complex (28) and known to produce lymphatic leukemia after an extended latent period (29), produces a rapid immunodepression without acute erythroleukemia. Thus, virus-induced immunodepression without transformation of target cells is apparently not sufficient for immediate production of neoplastic disease. It should be noted, however, that the great majority of these investigations have been studies of immune responsiveness to non-leukemic antigens; few, if any, examinations have been directed toward understanding the relationship of immunode-pression of the host's response to the leukemogenic virus, itself.

The participation of the cell mediated immune response in defense against virus-induced solid tumors has been con-vincingly demonstrated (30), but the importance of this re-sponse in murine leukemia viral infections has not been as well documented. Indeed, the results which have been report-ed are conflicting and confusing. Increased susceptibility to murine sarcoma virus (31) and tumor homografts (27,24) have been reported in FV infected mice, suggesting impairment of cell mediated immunity. Rejection of skin grafts across a relatively weak non-H2 histocompatibility barrier was found to be diminished in mice infected on the third day of life with Gross passage A leukemia virus (32). In contrast, graft vs. host reactivity in FV-infected mice was found to be normal by Snyder and Dory (24). Finally, infection with murine leukemia viruses have been shown to impair lymphocyte reactivity to antigens and non-specific mitogens as measured by both production of macrophage migration inhibitory factor (MIF) and stimulation in response to phytohemagglutinin or histoincompatible lymphocytes (33,34,19).

The participation of macrophage in immune and non-immune functions has been well documented(35,36,37,38). The macro-phage has been found to be an integral part of the cellular events that lead to both humoral antibody production to large antigens such as SRBCs (39) and to host resistance to viral infections (40,41,42). More recent studies have attributed increasing importance to macrophage participation in cell mediated immunity. Exposure of lymphocytes to macrophages in vitro increases the degree of lymphocyte stimulation by PHA (43) or specific antigens (44), and facilitates the in vitro allograft reaction (45).

Macrophages have been shown to participate in the host response to neoplastic disease (46,47,48,49). In addition, treatment of animals with reticuloendothelial system (RES) stimulants have been shown to enhance resistance of these animals to tumor transplants and oncogenic viruses (50,51,52, 53), whereas RES depressants have lowered host resistance to similar challenge (4,54,55,56). Finally, the neoplastic process, itself, has been shown to have varying effects on the RES, although, in general, increased RES activity has been correlated with a more favorable and decreased RES activity with a less favorable clinical course (3,4,57,58).

Finally, a major part of the adjuvant activity of agents which have been shown to enhance host resistance to neoplastic disease, such as BCG (51,59), Complete Freunds Adjuvant (CFA) (60), or pyran (61), has been reported to be mediated through specific activation of macrophages (53).

Reticuloendothelial system activity has been shown to be affected by FV infection (62) and peritoneal macrophages have been demonstrated to contain infective FV (63). It has furthermore been suggested by some investigators (13,21,22, 64) although denied by others (65,66) that the macrophage might play some role in FV induced immunodepression.

Since maturation of many host immune functions is dependent upon the integrity of specific lymphoid and macrophage cells, a defect in processing of antigen by one cell type or in cooperation between cells may lead to a cascade effect manifested by immuno-incompetence. Therefore, effective immunotherapy of cancer may require a precise identification of the specific impairment in cellular function of the host and restoration of this impaired function.

In our own work, we have attempted to cure virus-induced leukemia by restoring immunocompetence to infected animals. By identifying those immune and non-immune functions which are required for the suppression of murine leukemia, we hope to find ways to stimulate these functions selectively and apply such knowledge to the treatment of human leukemia.

In the murine leukemia model which we have developed for the study of restoration of immune and non-immunocompetence an established FV infection is produced in 100% of DBA/2 mice by the third day after virus inoculation as determined by viremia and the presence of leukemic cells in the spleen(67).

Mice begin to die on the 27th day and all mice are dead on the 74th day. A single inoculation of statolon, an extract of the mold Penicillium stoloniferum on the third day after virus inoculation completely suppresses the virulent leukemia viral infection in 40 to 90% of mice.

Statolon-treated mice with suppressed infections display no gross pathological, clinical or hemotological manifestations of leukemia for many months, but in some of these mice, FV emerges spontaneously late in life to produce characteristic FV leukemia indicating that the virus was present in the suppressed state during the prolonged clinical remission. Attempts to isolate infective FV from filtrates of the blood or spleen of these mice in which the disease has been suppressed by statolon have been unsuccessful, but transfer of their spleen cells in large numbers to normal mice produces FV leukemia from which the virus can be readily isolated. Interferon appears not to be the crucial defense mechanism involved in suppression of FV leukemia by statolon since interferon levels in mice which rapidly develop leukemia despite statolon treatment are as high as in mice which develop FV dormant infections (68). Analysis of the effect of statolon on FV replication and production of FV transformed spleen cells reveals that FV is cleared from the blood within 24 hours after statolon administration and that all cellular leukemogenic activity in the spleen disappears by the 38th day after inoculation (69). At that time the spleen contains many cells capable of inducing resistance to FV in normal mice (70). As these FV-resistance-inducing cells decrease in number during the subsequent 200 days, leukemogenic cells reappear and in some cases, characteristic FV leukemia develops.

Friend virus infected mice are immunosuppressed as shown by studies with non-leukemic antigens. Also FV virus-specific antibody cannot be found in leukemic mice. Statolon treatment of leukemic mice, however, induces antibody which neutralizes FV, passively agglutinates FV-coated SRBC, binds to and is cytotoxic for FV leukemic spleen cells and protects normal mice against FV infection (71). Mice treated with polyinosinic-polycytidylic acid (poly I:C) or Newcastle disease virus, or with antilymphocyte serum plus statolon, produce high titers of interferon and clear blood of Friend virus within 24 hours, but do not produce FV cytotoxic antibody and do not suppress the FV to a dormant state (72).

In order to study the role of humoral immunity in suppression of FV leukemia by statolon, we employed sheep erythrocytes (SRBC) as an antigenic challenge quantitating their antibody response by measuring anti-SRBC-plaque forming

cells (PFC) by the Jerne technique. We found that statolon
treatment rapidly restored humoral antibody competence to
SRBC in all leukemic mice, and all mice subsequently developed FV cytotoxic antibody (73). However, not all treated
mice entered clinical remissions and those mice that did
contained significantly higher levels of FV-cytotoxic antibody than did mice that became leukemic in spite of the
statolon treatment (74). A further lack of correlation between early restoration of humoral antibody production to
SRBC and suppression of FV leukemia was seen in experiments
with COAM, a chlorite oxidized oxyamylose. Administration
of COAM intraperitoneally 3 hours prior to statolon induced
more interferon and FV-cytotoxic antibody and a greater percentage of FV dormant infections than did statolon alone.
However, restoration of humoral immunity to SRBC to normal
levels was delayed in the COAM-statolon-treated group and
occurred long after FV cytotoxic antibody was produced (75).
Thus, while our hypothesis that humoral immunity is of prime
importance in suppression of FV leukemia was supported, the
experiments reveal that caution should be exercised in evaluating such immunity using non-leukemic antigens.

   We found that cell mediated responses as measured by
Concanavalin A stimulation of spleen cells was restored to
normal levels following treatment with statolon. We do not
know whether restoration of the Con A response to spleen
cells preceded suppression of FV leukemia and was requisite
for it or merely followed restoration of a clinically normal
state (76). Therefore, the role of cell mediated immunity
in suppression of FV leukemia by statolon remains to be
determined. Statolon may restore humoral immunocompetence
to leukemic mice by correcting a functional defect in "T"
cells since the humoral responses to both FV and SRBC are
believed to be "T" cell-dependent. In vitro experiments with
purified cell populations of lymphoid cells from untreated
and statolon-treated normal and FV-leukemic mice should
elucidate the role of these cell types in the suppression of
FV leukemia.

   Finally, we have found that peritoneal macrophages from
leukemic mice are suppressed in their ability to ingest
hemolysis-treated SRBC. Treatment of the leukemic macrophages with statolon both in vivo and in vitro restores the
phagocytic function of these leukemic macrophages to normal
levels (77). Macrophages probably play a significant role in
defense against FV leukemia as shown by the enhanced leukemogenesis following treatment of mice with silica, an agent
which is selectively toxic for macrophages (78). In addition,
the suppression of phagocytic function of peritoneal

macrophages from FV leukemic mice suggests that subversion of these cells may be requisite for leukemogenesis. The ability of statolon to restore normal levels of phagocytic function to leukemic macrophages in vitro indicates that restoration in vivo may be a crucial step in suppression of the disease.

In summary, then, we have found an agent that abrogates the immunodepressive effects of Friend leukemia virus, stimulates production of an FV cytotoxic antibody and completely suppresses established erythroleukemia. This agent, statolon, also restores other immune and non-immune functions of leukemic mice. We believe that an intensive study of this unique model focusing on the mechanisms involved in restoration of immune and non-immune competence to leukemic mice and characterization of the active fractions of statolon which restore such competence will provide important clues for infective immunotherapy of human leukemia.

This work was supported by Public Health Service Grant No. 5. R01 CA 12461-04

REFERENCES

1. Waldmann, T.A., Strober, W. and Blaese, R.M. (1972). Ann. Intern. Med. 77: 605.
2. Hersh, E.M., and Freireich, E.J.(1968). In: Methods in Cancer Research (H. Busch, ed.), Vol. 4: 355 Academic Press, New York.
3. Al-Sarraf, M., et al.(1970). Cancer 26: 262.
4. Harris, J.E., Ramesh Bagai and Stewart, T. (1971). Blood 38: 805.
5. Hersh, E.M., et al. (1971). New Eng. J. Med. 285: 1211
6. Moore, G.E. (1973). Prog. in Clin. Cancer 5: 107.
7. Yashphe, D.J. (1971). Israel J. Med. Sci. 7:90.
8. Hirsch, M.S., Black, P.H., and Proffitt, M.R. (1971). Fed. Proc. 30: 1852.
9. Burstein, N.A., and Allison, A.C. (1970). Nature 225:1139.
10. Nehlsen, S.L. (1971). Transplant. Proc. 3: 811.
11. Solnik, C., Gleichmann, H., Kavanah, M., and Schwartz, R.S. (1973). Cancer Res. 33: 2068.
12. Old, L.J., et al. (1960). Ann. N.Y. Acad. Sci. 88: 264.
13. Friedman, H. and Ceglowski, W.S. (1972). In:Prog. in Immunol. First Intl. Congr. Immunol.(B. Amos, ed.), p. 815. Academic Press, New York.

14. Wedderburn, N., and Salaman, M.H. (1968). Immunol. 15:439.
15. Ceglowski, W.S. and Friedman, H. (1970). J. Immunol. 105: 1406.
16. Salaman, M.H. (1970). Proc. Roy. Soc. Med. 63: 11.
17. Bennett, M., and Steeves, R.A. (1970). J. Natl. Cancer Inst. 44: 1107.
18. Häyry, P., et.al.(1970). J. Nat. Cancer Inst. 44: 1311.
19. Mortensen, R.F., Ceglowski, W.S. and Friedman, H. (1973). J. Immunology 111: 1810.
20. Dent, P.B. (1972). Prog. Med. Virol. 14:1.
21. Odaka, T., et.al. (1966). Japan. J. Exptl. Med. 36: 277.
22. Salaman, M.H. (1969). Antibiotic Chem., NY 15: 393.
23. Ceglowski, W.S. and Friedman, H. (1969). Nature 224: 1318.
24. Schneider, M. and Doré, J.F. (1969). Rev. Franc. ET. Clin. Biol. 14: 1010.
25. Borella, L. (1969). J. Immunology 103: 185.
26. Seidel, H.J. and Lauenstein, K. (1969). Z. Krebsforsch. 72: 219.
27. Deodhar, S.D. and Chiang, T. (1970). Fed. Proc. 29: 560.
28. Rowson, K.E.K. and Parr, I.B. (1970). Intl. J. Cancer 5: 96.
29. Carter, R.L., et. al. (1970). Intl. J. Cancer 6: 290.
30. Gaugas, J.M., et. al. (1973). Br. J. Cancer 27: 10.
31. Chirigos, M.A., et. al. (1968). Cancer Res. 28: 1055.
32. Dent, P.B., et.al. (1965). Proc. Soc. Exptl. Biol. Med. 119: 869.
33. Borella, L. (1972). J. Immunol. 108: 45.
34. Friedman, H. and Ceglowski, W.S. (1971). Proc. Soc. Exptl. Biol. Med. 136: 154.
35. Nelson, D.S. (1969). Macrophages and Immunity, North Holland Publ. Col., Amsterdam.
36. Pearsall, N.N. and Weiser, R.S. (1970). The Macrophage. Lea and Febiger, Philadelphia.
37. Unanue, E.R. (1972). Adv. Immunol 15: 95.
38. Vernon-Roberts, B. (1972). The Macrophage. Cambridge University Press, Cambridge, Great Britain.
39. Cruchaud, A. and Unanue, E.R. (1971). J. Immunol. 107: 1329.
40. Allison, A.C.(1970). In: Mononuclear Phagocytes. (Van Furth, R., ed.) p. 442, F.A. Davis Co., Philadelphia.
41. Mims, C.A. (1964). Bacteriol. Rev. 28:30.
42. Panijel, J. and Cayeux, P. (1968). Immunol. 14: 769.
43. Levis, W.R. and Robbins, J.H. (1970). Exp. Cell. Res. 61: 153.
44. Seeger, R.C. and Oppenheim, J.J. (1970). J. Exp. Med.132: 44.

45. Lonai, P. and Feldman, M. (1971). Immunol. 21: 861.
46. Cruse, J.M. et.al. (1973). Transplant. Proc. V: 961.
47. Evans, R. et.al. (1973). Proc. Soc. Exptl. Biol. Med. 143: 256.
48. Hibbs, Jr., J.B. (1973) Science 180: 868.
49. Kramer, J.J. and Granger, G.A. (1972). Cell. Immunol. 3: 88.
50. Diller, I.C. et.al. (1963). Cancer Res. 23:201.
51. Hirsch, M.S. et.al. (1972). J. Immunol. 108: 1312.
52. Munson, A.E. el.al. (1972). Cancer Res. 32: 1397.
53. Taub, R.N. (1970). Progr. Allergy 14: 208.
54. Bailiff, R.N. (1956). Cancer Res. 16: 479.
55. Ghose, T. (1957). Indian J. Med. Sci. 11: 900.
56. Zarling, J.M. and Tevethia, S.S. (1973). J. Nat. Cancer Inst. 50: 149.
57. Groch, G.S. et.al. (1965). Blood 26: 489.
58. Pisano, J.C. et.al. (1973). Proc. Soc. Exp. Biol. Med. 142: 1355.
59. Mackaness, G.B. (1970). In: Infectious Agents and Host Reactions. (Mudd, Stuart, ed.), p. 61, W.B. Saunders Co., Philadelphia.
60. Hibbs, J.B., Jr. et.al. (1972). Proc. Soc. Exp. Biol. Med. 139: 1053.
61. Regelson, W. and Munson, A.E. (1970). Ann. N.Y. Acad. Sci. 173: 831.
62. Gledhill, A.W. et.al. (1965). Br. J. Exp. Path. 46: 433.
63. Odaka, T. and Köhler, K. (1965). Zeitschr. Naturforsch. 206: 473.
64. Ceglowski, W.S. and Friedman, H. (1968). J. Immunol. 101: 594.
65. Dracott, B.N. et.al. (1972). J. Gen. Virol. 14: 77.
66. Bendinelli, M. (1968). Immunol. 14: 837.
67. Wheelock, E.F., Caroline, N.L. and Moore, R.D. (1969). J. Virol. 4: 1.
68. Wheelock, E.F. and Caroline, N.L. (1970). Proc. Intl. Symp. Interferon, Lyon .
69. Wheelock, E.F., Caroline, N.L. and Moore, R.D. (1971). J. Nat. Cancer Inst. 46: 797.
70. Wheelock, E.F. and Caroline, N.L. (1970). Ann. N.Y. Acad. Sci. 173: 582.
71. Wheelock, E.F., Toy, S.T., Caroline, N., et.al. (1972). J. Nat. Cancer Inst. 48: 665.
72. Toy, S.T., Weislow, O.S. and Wheelock, E.F. (1973). Proc. Soc. Exp. Biol. Med. 143: 726.
73. Weislow, O.S., Friedman, H. and Wheelock, E.F. (1973). Proc. Soc. Exp. Biol. Med. 142: 401.

74. Wheelock, E.F., Weislow, O.S. and Toy, S.T. (1973). In:
    Virus Tumorigenesis and Immunogenesis. (Ceglowski, W.S.
    and Friedman, H., eds.), p. 351, Academic Press, N.Y.
75. Weislow, O.S. and Wheelock, E.F. Infection & Immunity, in
    press.
76. Toy, S.T. and Wheelock, E.F. Cellular Immunology, in press.
77. Wheelock, E.F., Toy, S.T., Weislow, O.S. and Levy, M.H.
    (1974). In: Progress in Experimental Tumor Research.
    (Richards, V., ed.), Vol. 19, p. 369, S. Karger, Basel.
78. Larson, C.L. et.al. (1972). J. Nat. Cancer Inst. 48: 1403.

4

Does Immunity Promote or Inhibit Tumor Growth?

Richmond T. Prehn

Most chemically-induced tumors exhibit, by transplantation tests, strong tumor associated antigens capable of arousing a specific immune response. Under proper conditions this response can inhibit tumor growth even in syngeneic (genetically identical) animals. However, a weak and/or early imimune response can stimulate tumor growth. This is a positive stimulation, not just a blocking of the resistance reaction. In general, each tumor is immunologically specific when tested by transplantation tests and cross reactivity is rare unless there has been a superimposed viral infection. However, apparent cross reactivity is commonly demonstrated by a variety of in vitro tests.

The fact of immunostimulation and a variety of data of other kinds suggest that immunosurveillance is seldom an important influence on tumor incidence. On the contrary, the immune response may, as far as neoplasia is concerned, do more harm than good.

The modern revival of tumor immunology as a respectable discipline stemmed from the observation that even syngeneic mice could be successfully immunized against the growth of chemically-induced transplanted tumors. In the classical technique, a number of syngeneic mice were inoculated with the tumor to be tested; after a short period of growth the tumor implants were excised. After a rest period of a few days, the now presumptively immune mice were challenged with a second inoculation of the same tumor and the resulting growths compared with suitable controls. The almost invariable result was relatively poor growth in the immunized mice. Various types of controls established the tumor-specific nature of the immunity.

As the result of much work the following points about the immunology of chemically-induced tumors were established:

1. Each tumor is, by this test, individually specific. Even two tumors induced by the same methods in one and the same mouse usually fail to cross react, unless there is a superimposed viral infection.

2. While almost all tumors exhibit the phenomenon, the degree of immunogenicity varies markedly from tumor to tumor. Some, but probably not all of this variation may be due to the induction by some of the tumors of humoral "blocking factors" capable of interfering with cellular immunity.

3. There is a marked correlation between the latent period of the primary tumor and the apparent immunogenicity of the subsequent transplanted tumor generations. In general, those tumors that had been induced rapidly exhibit stronger immunogenicities than do those which originally appeared after a long latent period. In this connection, it is noteworthy that spontaneous tumors, which might be thought of as having very long average latencies, usually have little or no demonstrable immunogenicity by this transplantation test.

4. The correlation of latent period with immunogenicity disappears if the tumors are induced in immunologically depressed mice or in immunity-free environments (i.e., within diffusion chambers). The relatively high immunogenicities of those tumors with short latent periods is therefore probably due in part to immunoselection. It is known that the immune response is depressed by chemical oncogens, and therefore those tumors that arise early.during the period of maximal influence of the carcinogen on the immune response are permitted a higher average immunogenicity.

It must be emphasized that the preceding points were
established by an in vivo transplantation test. Somewhat
different conclusions may be reached if other test method-
ologies are used, in particular various in vitro tests of
tumor antigenicity. For example, it has been reported that
of lymphocytes from immunized mice are placed in contact
with carcinogen-induced syngeneic bladder tumor cells growing
in culture, an immune cytotoxic reaction occurs. By this
test, the immune lymphoid cells attack all bladder tumors,
i.e., there is complete cross reactivity among the individual
chemically-induced tumors. Other types of target cells are
spared so there is some type of specificity involved. Despite the fact that this in vitro test shows extensive cross
reactivity among the tumors, the classical transplantation
type of test reveals the tumors to be individually specific,
i.e., no cross reactivity can be detected. It is therefore
apparent that the in vivo and in vitro tests measure different phenomena--the in vivo may be more indicative of
significant physiological or pathological events.

The individual specificities of the chemically induced
tumors, as revealed by the transplantation type of test,
gives rise to the question of how many tumor types there
may be. Dr. Basombrio in my laboratory has filled in a
10 x 10 grid, i.e., he has tested each of ten tumors against
each of the others, both as immunizer and challenger, and
failed to find a reproducible cross reactivity. On the
other hand, cross reactions, and particularly partial cross
reactions, are occasionally seen. Thus, the number of types
is large -- probably in excess of 50 -- but it is certainly
not infinite.

The tumor associated transplantation antigens that I have
been discussing are undoubtedly surface antigens closely
related to the ordinary histocompatibility antigens. Little
progress has been made at their chemical characterization.
Recently it has been found that they may be present in the
circulation of tumor bearing animals, so progress in this
area may be rapid.

These are the principal characteristics of tumor-associ-
ated antigens, but what about their biological significance?
To be sure the reason why tumor cells have antigens of the
transplantation type is not known. One possible explanation
is that new antigens do not appear to be a necessary condition of the tumorous state. They are usually demonstrable,
but there are some rare tumors in which transplantation type
antigens are not detectable by any presently available test.
One would think that there would be strong selection favoring no or minimal antigenicity, and the fact already

61

mentioned, that spontaneous tumors arouse virtually no immune resistance might be a manifestation of such selection. Perhaps, as the theory of immunological surveillance tells us, spontaneous tumors represent a very small selected subpopulation that escaped the more usual suppression by immune surveillance precisely because of their lack of immunogenicity. (Whether their lack of immunogenicity by the transplantation test is due to lack of antigens or to blocking factors or both is not clear, but is irrelevant to the present argument).

If spontaneous tumors lack immunogenicity because they represent a small highly selected part of the total of transformational events, it follows that tumors that arise in the absence of any immune reaction, and thus do not undergo immunoselection, should be highly immunogenic. We tested this hypothesis by testing the immunogenicities of those tumors that arise "spontaneously" during tissue culture or among cells in diffusion chambers. Rather to our surprise, such tumors lacked immunogenicity, by the in vivo transplantation test. However, if a chemical carcinogen had been used, the tumors that arose among cells in tissue culture or in diffusion chambers were highly immunogenic. The conclusion was inescapable that tumors lack immunogenicity if a carcinogen is not overtly involved in their etiology, whether or not there is any possibility of an immune reaction. Spontaneous tumors lack immunogenicity, not because of immunoselection, but because the initial transformation did not involve a chemical agent (or virus) to any gross extent.

If spontaneous tumors in general do not arouse an appreciable resistance reaction (and this cannot be attributed to immunological surveillance), it is difficult to see what role the immune reaction plays. Perhaps surveillance is an effective force only in the case of those highly immunogenic tumors that are created by the application of large doses of chemical oncogens or highly selected laboratory viruses. In other words, immunological surveillance may be a laboratory artifact.

Although induced immune resistance to tumor growth is virtually undetectable in most spontaneous tumors, there may be a very little, almost subliminal, amount of such resistance. Is it possible that such a small reaction might be adequate for the purposes of surveillance? Perhaps a very small reaction could cope with the very few cells in a nascent tumor. If so, immunological surveillance might still be an effective force.

The relative effectiveness of immunity in relation to the number of tumor cells can be tested by simply titrating the size of an antigenic tumor inoculum in specifically immune animals and measuring the subsequent tumor growth. When such an experiment is performed, a surprising phenomenon is often, but not always, observed. Large numbers of tumor cells will usually overwhelm the immunity and grow despite it; somewhat smaller numbers are often completely inhibited; the surprising finding is that very small numbers may again show some growth. In other words, the titration curve is often biphasic; very small and very large inocula grow while those of intermediate size are inhibited. The growth of very small inocula is called "sneaking through" and is thought to be due to a delay in the afferent signal to the immune mechanism. This gives the tumor time to establish itself and begin to grow. Once growing, it becomes, for unknown reasons, much less vulnerable. Although the "sneaking through" phenomenon is often subtle and difficult to demonstrate, it has been observed in many laboratories (1). Its existence would seem to rule out the hypothesis that a very few tumor cells, as in a nascent tumor, might be unusually vulnerable to immunological surveillance.

The argument can now be summarized as follows: Spontaneous tumors as a class arouse little or no immune resistance to their growth; this lack is not a result of immune selection; and whatever little resistance they may arouse could not, judging by the evidence of the "sneaking through" phenomenon, cope with a nascent tumor. Therefore, immunological surveillance is not effective in spontaneous tumor systems.

Perhaps the reader will react to the above argument by citing the vast literature from both man and mouse to the effect that oncogenesis is more prevalent in conditions of immunodepression. However, all of the animal data relate to tumor induction with chemicals or with laboratory selected viruses which produce highly immunogenic tumors. Perhaps in such systems there is surveillance, although an alternative explanation of these data will be offered shortly. The data from immunodeficiency states in man concerning spontaneous tumors does not support the surveillance hypothesis. Although tumor incidence is indeed increased in such states, most, if not all, of the increment is due to tumors of the lymphoreticular system. If the increase were due to a lack of immunological surveillance, all types of tumors would be indiscriminately increased, not just tumors of the deficient or damaged organ.

Although the preceding argument could be regarded as conclusive, the best evidence against the theory of immunological surveillance is provided by the "nude" mouse. This animal is congenitally athymic. As a consequence, it will accept foreign skin grafts from virtually any source indefinitely. It should therefore have no capacity to "survey" for "foreign" tumor antigens. If the theory of immunological surveillance were correct, these animals, without any defense should have a very high tumor incidence. At the present time "nude" mice are still surviving in my germ-free colony after one year of age and as yet there have been no spontaneous tumors other than those of lymphoreticular origin. Under the conditions in which the "nude" mice are raised, i.e., germ-free, the presence or absence of an effective immune capacity against foreign antigenic tissues does not determine the tumor incidence or even influence it significantly. Of course, if these animals were exposed to any of the laboratory oncogenic viruses the outcome would probably be different, although we have not yet done the experiment.

If immunological surveillance is effective only in unusual circumstances, i.e., exposure to high levels of oncogenic viruses or chemical oncogens, does the immune reaction play any role at all in the biology of ordinary spontaneous tumors, those tumors with little immunogenic potential? It is, in my opinion, highly probable that it does, but it is not the role usually envisioned.

Several years ago a controversial body of literature suggested that a minor genetic disparity between mother and offspring, and a consequent mild immune reaction, might result in larger placentae and bigger and more numerous young (1). If this data were correct, the implication was clear that a mild immune reaction might stimulate rather than inhibit the growth of target cells. If the immune reaction could stimulate the growth of a mildly antigenic fetus, might it not do the same for a mildly antigenic tumor?

This immunostimulation hypothesis was tested, in the first instance, by mixing immune spleen cells with target tumor cells in varying ratios and placing the mixtures subcutaneously in immunologically depressed mice. It was found that, just as predicted, low ratios of immune cells stimulated the growth of the tumor cells, as compared with the effect of control non-immune spleen cells. High ratios gave the anticipated inhibition. Essentially similar results have been obtained in completely in vitro tests and the results have found confirmation in several laboratories (2).

Recently, Dr. Jeejeebhoy, working in my laboratory, has shown that the "immune" cells obtained from the peripheral blood of mice shortly after (five days) tumor implantation were stimulatory to the tumor in an in vitro test, while equal numbers were inhibitory after a longer interval (3). It thus appears that whenever the immune response is weak, as it must be early in the course of tumor growth, or when the tumor has little immunogenicity, the effect is stimulation.

We are therefore faced with a biphasic immune effect and the net result will depend upon a complex equation relating tumor immunogenicity, and intrinsic growth potential. Perhaps, as the "nude" mouse may yet reveal, the total absence of immunity may result in fewer spontaneous tumors than will an ineffective level of immune "surveillance"!

We can now return to the original question concerning the biological function of tumor associated antigens. Their variation in amount, specificity and effectiveness in different tumors and their possible complete absence in some rare instances suggests that these antigens are not directly and intimately linked to the tumorous state. The fact that they are associated to a marked degree with the rapid oncogenesis of a chemical agent, even under conditions in which no immune selection can occur suggests that they are, in the case of the chemicals, chance phenomena which are more likely to occur in a transformed cell if the impetus to transformation, and thus the number of transformational events, is large. Since a tumor can to a considerable degree, by modulation and/or selection, alter its immunogenicity, it is probable that there is a selective tendency favoring tumors with an immunogenicity within the stimulatory range -- this may be a high degree of immunogenicity in the animal depressed by oncogen or other agent and a very low degree in the case of spontaneous tumors arising in normal mice.

From what has been said it is obvious that even in the case of highly immunogenic chemically induced tumors, the higher incidence resulting from immunodepression may not be evidence of the ordinary efficacy of surveillance, but rather evidence that the level of immune reactivity has been reduced to a more stimulatory range. Immunostimulation may also underlie the "sneaking through" phenomenon previously discussed.

The mechanisms of stimulation are unknown. There is some evidence, from other laboratories, that it can be mediated by "T" cells (4) and other evidence that it cannot be mediated by macrophages (5). Stimulation can be produced by low levels of specific antibody as well as by low levels of lymphotoxin.

The fact that the immune response can be either stimulatory or inhibitory to target cells depending upon circumstances suggests that it plays a regulatory rather than a merely defensive role. It certainly did not evolve in order to stimulate tumor growth; this must be a perversion of some related normal activity. The recently developing evidence that lymphoid cells have the potential to react against "self" as well as "non-self" suggests a role for the lymphoid system in normal growth regulation--certainly a very old idea. In our laboratory Dr. Michael Pliskin has been gathering evidence that the lymphoid system may play a role in liver regeneration. This sort of investigation may prove very instructive in the years to come.

The very fact that immunosurveillance may be less effective than was generally believed offers an opportunity that would not otherwise have existed. A highly efficient surveillance mechanism would mean that there was little hope of improving the situation by any type of immunotherapy, but an inefficient mechanism may possibly be augmented. However, the existence of immunostimulation as well as immunoinhibition of target tumor cells means that attempts at immunotherapy may be even more hazardous than was already apparent. The possibility of doing harm by altering the immune mechanism to a stimulatory level of activity is very real and has probably already occurred in some instances. It seems that a much better methodology for assessing the level of the host's immune responsiveness to his tumor is required before immunotherapy can be put on a rational scientific basis.

This investigation was supported by Public Health Service Research Grant Nos. CA-08856, CA-06927, CA-05255, CA-13456, RR-05539 from the National Institutes of Health, and by an appropriation from the Commonwealth of Pennsylvania.

REFERENCES

1. Prehn, R.T., and Lappé, M.A.(1971).Transplant Rev.7: 26.
2. Prehn, R.T. (1972). Science 176: 170.
3. Jeejeebhoy, H. (1974). Intl. J. Cancer 13: 665.
4. Fidler, I.J. (1974). Cancer Research 34: 491.
5. Fidler, I.J. (1973). J. Natl. Can. Inst. 50: 1307.

5

Immune Response-Pathogenicity of Viral Infection
Diane Griffin

The role of the immune response in the pathogenesis of most viral infections is largely unknown. Delineating this role is dependent on an understanding of the biologic properties of the particular virus under study and on an understanding of what types of immune responses are evoked. When these basic parameters have been determined, the consequences of the interaction between the viral infection and the immune responses to the infection may be studied.

TYPES OF VIRAL INFECTION

There are many different groups of viruses which vary in the cells they can infect and in the effects that they have on those cells. The outcome of the infection of a cell with a virus is dependent on the particular biologic nature of the virus as well as the nature of the cell infected (1,2). For instance, a virus may infect a cell and cause lysis of that cell (lytic viruses such as poliovirus), the virus may become integrated and transform the cell (oncogenic viruses such as SV40), or the virus may cause no discernible damage to the cell (noncytopathic viruses such as lymphocytic choriomeningitis virus). The mechanism of spread of a given virus to other susceptible cells may be by lysis of the cell

with release of infectious particles into the extracellular
space (picornaviruses such as poliovirus), by budding of
virus from the cell surface into the extracellular space
(myxoviruses such as influenza) or by spread from infected
cells to an adjacent noninfected cell without entering the
extracellular space (herpesviruses such as herpes simplex
virus). The type of viral release may determine whether
newly-formed virus is accessible or inaccessible to neutralization by antibody. Some virus infections may result in the
production of large amounts of viral antigen but very little
infectious virus (defective infections such as subacute
sclerosing panencephalitis)(3). Finally, most viurses are
composed of a number of complex antigens which in many instances have not yet been defined. Certain groups of viruses
such as those surrounded by an envelope (i.e., myxoviruses)
insert viral antigens into the host cell membrane before budding off from that membrane (1). Other viruses, particularly
the oncogenic viruses, code for new antigens on the cell surface which are not structural components of the virus (2).
Each of these viral antigens may induce a specific immune
response.

IMMUNE RESPONSES

   The immune response to any particular viral antigen may
take a number of forms depending on the nature of the antigen and how it is presented to the immune system of the host.
The two categories of immune response which are generally
recognized are cellular (mediated by T cells) and humoral
(mediated by B cells). There are many components of the possible immune responses to the viral antigens presented during
an infection. The cell-mediated immune response produces
lymphocytic cells sensitized to viral antigens. These antigens may be internal or external components of the virus or
may be antigens expressed only on the surface of an infected
cell. Sensitized lymphocytic cells may have a number of biologically important capabilities (4): 1) Sensitized cells
may be cytotoxic and may damage a viral antigen-bearing cell,
exposing any internal infectious virus to neutralization by
antibody. If the infection is noncytopathic the cytotoxic
lymphoid cell may damage a cell which would not have been
harmed by the virus infection alone. 2) Sensitized cells may
also be capable of proliferating after reexposure to the sensitizing viral antigen. This blastogenic response serves to
increase the number of virus-sensitized cells. 3) Sensitized
cells may produce a number of soluble factors which directly

influence macrophages. A chemotactic substance may bring phagocytic cells into the area of viral replication. A migration inhibitory factor may keep them in the area and a macrophage activating factor may make the macrophages capable of more rapid phagocytosis and destruction of certain organisms. 5) Sensitized cells may also produce interferon or antibody locally.

The humoral immune (antibody) response may be directed against any or all of the viral antigens. The biologic properties of the antibody are determined by the antigen to which it is directed and by the class of immunoglobulin (IgM, IgG, IgA, etc.) which is synthesized. Neutralizing antibody is probably directed against that portion of the viral coat responsible for attachment to cell receptors and serves to prevent infection of other cells. Antibody may also be formed to interior components of the virus and play no role in preventing infection of other cells. Antibody may be formed to antigens expressed only on the cell surface. Such antibody, if capable of fixing complement(cytotoxic antibody) may destroy an infected cell before it has released infectious virus into the surrounding milieu of susceptible cells. Cytotoxic antibody could also destroy a cell which might not have been destroyed by the virus itself. In addition a non-cytotoxic antibody could theoretically block the action of a cytotoxic lymphocyte by binding preferentially to the cell surface. Additionally soluble viral antigen-antibody complexes may be formed, and in situations where the viral infection is persistent and large amounts of antigen are continuously released into the circulation the entire additional spectrum of immune complex disease can be produced (5,6).

Finally, one of the host cells that the virus infects may be a part of the immune system itself. Such an interaction could produce a viral-induced impairment or enhancement of the immune response (7). Impairment would occur if the virus destroyed or functionally incapacitated the lymphoid cell responsible for induction of the immune response, antibody formation, or cellular effector mechanism. Enhancement could occur if the lymphoid cell were not harmed but responded immunologically to the viral antigen or proliferated after infection. Such viral-induced alterations could occur in cells involved in either or both humoral or cellular immune responses.

RESPONSES TO A SPECIFIC VIRUS

Given these multifaceted problems it seemed most reasona-
ble to study one viral infection and its immune response in
some depth. The viral infection chosen for study in the
laboratory of Dr. Richard Johnson was Sindbis virus infection
of the mouse. Sindbis virus is the prototype of the group A
arboviruses and causes a mild febrile illness in man after
natural exposure (8). Sindbis virus has a lipoprotein envelope which is acquired as it buds from the surface of the
infected cell which is subsequently lysed by this infection.
In the suckling (1-2 day) mouse it causes a fatal encephalitis, but in the weanling (4 week) mouse Sindbis virus infection causes a non-fatal encephalitis when inoculated intracerebrally or a local myositis when inoculated subcutaneously. The sites of viral replication (the brain or muscle) are
characterized histologically by a marked perivascular infil-
trate of mononuclear cells which begins 3-4 days after infection, peaks at 7-8 days and then subsides between 10 and
21 days. Following infection the animal is immune to reinfection for a prolonged period (9,10).

The basic parameters of the events during typical nonfatal
Sindbis virus encephalitis in the weanling mouse are as
follows: the virus is cytolytic and replicates rapidly in
the brain. Infectious virus is produced and can be titered
by plaque formation on chick embryo fibroblasts within 24
hours. Maximum virus growth is at 3 days, and by 7 days
Sindbis virus has been eliminated from the brain (Fig. 1).
Neutralizing antibody is detectable in the serum of infected
mice by 3 days, peaks at 6-7 days and then plateaus. Mice
do not appear ill during the course of this infection.

In attempting to determine the role of the immune response
in recovery from this infection attention was first focused
on the nature of the perivascular inflammatory cells (11).
1) What type of cells are they? 2) Where do they come from?
3) What brought them there? 4) What role do they have in the
disease? Morphologically the cells are mononuclear, but that
does not allow differentiation of lymphocytes from macrophages. Macrophages are by definition phagocytic cells and
can be distinguished from lymphocytes by this property. To
determine whether the cells were macrophages or lymphocytes,
animals were injected intravenously with the particulate dye
India ink. Those cells taking up the dye can be identified
as phagocytic. India ink given 4 days after virus and 1 hour
before sacrifice labels blood monocytes, but none of the
cells in the established cerebral inflammatory response.
However, if the Sindbis virus-infected mouse is examined 24

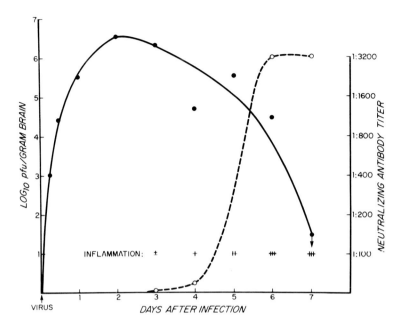

Fig. 1. Virus multiplication in brains of weanling mice
(●————●), development of serum neutralizing antibody (●- - -●)
and inflammation after intracerebral inoculation with Sindbis
virus.

---

hours after ink injection, labeled cells are readily identified distant from as well as around the cerebral blood vessels. These results demonstrate that many of the cells which
appear morphologically to be lymphocytes are really committed
macrophages prior to entering the inflammatory reaction and
that the cells are derived from the blood rather than from
the brain since cells are exposed to and can ingest the ink
only while in circulation.

These animals can also be studied by inoculating them with
tritiated thymidine (^{3}H-Tdr) (11) which will label new DNA
being synthesized and therefore will label dividing cells.
Which cells are labeled can then be determined by autoradio-
graphy. If ^{3}H-Tdr is given frequently after intracerebral
virus inoculation, 90% of the perivascular mononuclear cells
are labeled and less than 25% of the mononuclear cells in
the peripheral blood are labeled. If ^{3}H-Tdr is given before
virus inoculation more than 50% of the mononuclear cells were
labeled in the perivascular infiltrates developing 3-6 days

later. If animals were given ^{3}H-Tdr after virus inoculation and sacrificed 1 hour later, no cells in the peripheral blood were labeled but 10% of the cerebral inflammatory cells were. Results of the ^{3}H-Tdr labeling indicated that 1) the majority of cells in the inflammatory response are derived from the blood; 2) the cells are derived selectively from a population of short-lived mononuclear cells and 3) the cells do not divide in the blood but start dividing actively after entering the perivascular reaction.

The factors which initiate the immigration of these cells into the perivascular spaces of an infected animal are undoubtedly complex. It has been traditionally thought that the inciting factor was nonspecific and dependent on destruction of virus-infected cells (12,13). An alternative hypothesis was that this mononuclear inflammatory response was analogous to the tuberculin reaction and was immunologically specific. One objection to the latter hypothesis was that the infiltration begins 3-4 days after virus is first inoculated. This was considered somewhat rapid for a traditional delayed hypersensitivity or cell-mediated immune response.

IS INFLAMMATORY RESPONSE TO VIRAL INFECTION IMMUNOLOGICALLY SPECIFIC?

Experiments were designed to answer the question of whether the induction of the inflammatory response was immunologically specific or nonspecific (14). Weanling inbred BALB/c mice were inoculated intracerebrally with Sindbis virus and 24 hours later they were given 250 mg/kg cyclophosphamide for immunosuppression. Cyclophosphamide is an alkylating agent which inhibits cellular DNA synthesis and therefore cellular replication. The cells most affected by this drug are those dividing rapidly, primarily the phagocytic monocytes, other bone marrow cells, and intestinal lining cells. In addition to these cells which always have a rapid turnover, a burst of cellular division is induced in cells of the lymphoid system within 24 hours of antigenic stimulation. The cells dividing are those immunologically competent cells which are responding to the antigenic challenge and thus are selectively destroyed by this immunosuppressive regimen.

The consequences of suppressing the immune response to a viral infection are dependent on the individual virus-host relationship. In the case of Sindbis virus encephalitis in the weanling mouse viral growth was not enhanced and mice did not die, but instead virus growth persisted well beyond day 7 when in the non-immunosuppressed mouse viral clearance would have been complete (Fig. 2). Viral clearance occurred about day 13-14 when the effects of immunosuppression were

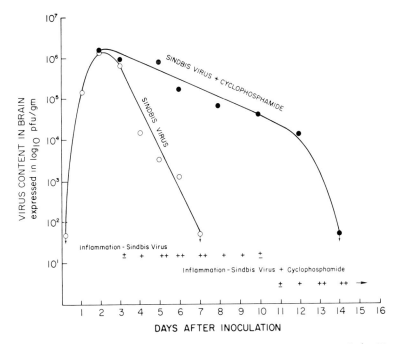

Fig. 2. Virus multiplication and development of inflammation in brains of weanling mice after intracerebral inoculation with Sindbis virus. Persistence of virus and delay in
the inflammatory response are shown in mice receiving cyclophosphamide 24 hours after virus (from McFarland, Griffin &
Johnson, 1973). Reprinted with permission from Rockefeller
University.

waning and antibody appeared. Brains of these immunosuppressed mice examined on day 8 showed no inflammatory response and provided a model for determining what cellular
and/or serum components were necessary for the perivascular
infiltration of monocytes. Was it necessary to replace only
the phagocytic mononuclear cells or were specifically sensitized immunologically competent cells also necessary? What
role did antibody have? Adoptive immunization with cells
and/or serum was used to answer these questions.

METHODS

The Sindbis virus-infected, cyclophosphamide-suppressed
mice were the recipients. Donor mice were prepared by inocu-

lating Sindbis virus or control tissue culture fluid subcutaneously into the footpads. Subsequently these mice were bled for immune or control serum. Local lymph nodes draining the sites of virus replication were taken for a source of immune or control lymph node cells. Bone marrow was taken as a source of monocytes. Transfer of cells and/or serum was done on day 3 after Sindbis virus inoculation (2nd day after cyclophosphamide) and the animals examined on day 8. Only those transfers which included Sindbis-sensitized lymph node cells were capable of reconstituting the inflammatory response. This response was amplified by any (immune or nonimmune) source of monocytes, but monocytes alone, even from Sindbis-sensitized animals could not reconstitute the response (Fig. 3). Likewise, Sindbis immune serum did not reconstitute the inflammatory response even when combined with nonimmune lymph node cells and/or any monocyte source. It was concluded that the induction of the inflammatory response in this viral encephalitis was immunologically specific.

The time needed to develop sensitized lymphocytes in Sindbis virus-infected mice can be determined by using an in vitro method for measuring cell-mediated immunity. There are a number of in vitro methods currently available for assessing cell-mediated immunity (15) and most can be adapted for use with viral antigens. 1) The inhibition of macrophage migration is a test which depends on the fact that sensitized lymphocytes produce a macrophage migration inhibition factor (MIF) when exposed to the sensitizing antigen. MIF inhibits the migration of macrophages from any source. In one common version of the test sensitized or·control lymphocytes are mixed with macrophages in a capillary tube and exposed to the test antigen. This antigen may be viral in nature. The area of migration of the macrophages under test and control situations can then be quantitated and a measure of cellular

Fig. 3. Horizontal sections of mouse brains 8 days after intracerebral inoculation of Sindbis virus. Sections show normal inflammatory response to virus (a), ablation of the response by a single dose of cyclophosphamide given 24 hours after virus;(b), reconstitution of the response with Sindbis virus-sensitized lymph node cells and bone marrow cells given 48 hours after cyclophosphamide;(c), and lack of reconstitution of the response with control tissue culture antigen-sensitized lymph node and bone marrow cells;(d). Hematoxylin and eosin. X34. (from McFarland, Griffin & Johnson, 1972). Reprinted with permission from Rockefeller University.

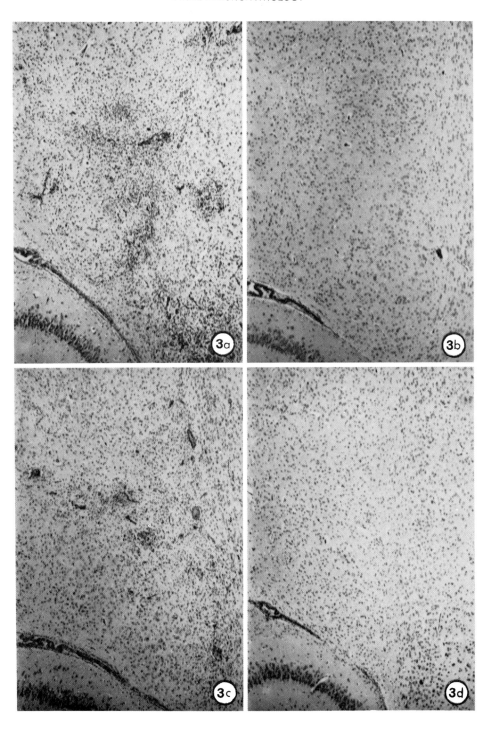

immunity obtained. 2) Lymphocyte cytotoxicity measures the
killing of target cells by lymphocytes sensitized to a component of the target cell membrane. The cytotoxicity can be
quantitated by counting dead cells or live cells remaining or
by measuring the release of an incorporated radioactive iso-
tope such as ^{51}CR or ^{125}I-iododeoxyuridine from the damaged
target cells. To use the cytotoxicity test in viral systems
the virus antigen must be incorporated into the target cell
membrane either by using a line of chronically infected cells
(carrier culture) or by using acutely infected cells at a
time when viral antigen is expressed on the surface, but before cell lysis by the virus occurs. The percent of target
cells killed by sensitized lymphocytes over control lymphocytes is a measure of the cytotoxicity of the sensitized
lymphocyte population. 3) Lymphocyte transformation is a test
which measures the proliferative response of a sensitized
cell when it is exposed again to the sensitizing antigen.
Lymphocyte transformation is usually quantitated by measuring
the incorporation of radioactive thymidine (^{3}H-Tdr) into
cellular DNA in the presence and absence of the sensitizing
antigen. Application of this test for measurement of lymphocyte sensitization to viral antigens must take into consider-
ation the numerous interactions which may influence the outcome. If the virus being used as antigen is capable of infecting the lymphocyte this interaction may result in impaired DNA synthesis or lysis of the lymphocytes. In this
instance inactivated virus would be a better antigen for the
test. Alternatively it is possible that viral infection of
the lymphocyte may stimulate DNA synthesis such as some
tumor viruses do in other cell systems, or it may have no
nonimmunologic effect on the lymphocyte. The amount of ^{3}H-
Tdr incorporated into DNA of sensitized cells in the presence
of antigen as opposed to control antigen is a measure of
cellular immunity.

Lymphocytes can also be stimulated to divide nonspecifi-
cally by certain substances known as mitogens which attach to
glycoproteins on the lymphocyte surface. Phytohemagglutinin
and concanavalin A are mitogens which specifically stimulate
T lymphocytes (16). Bacterial lipopolysaccharides (endotoxins) stimulate B cell precursors (17). Pokeweed mitogen
can stimulate B and T cells (18). Transformation to specific
antigens may also involve DNA synthesis by either or both B
and T cells (19).

Lymphocyte transformation was chosen as the test system
for studies with lymphocytes from Sindbis virus-infected animals (20). Adult mice were infected by inoculation of Sindbis virus into all footpads. At appropriate times after

76

infection the draining lymph nodes (popliteal, brachial and axillary) and spleens were removed to test for lymphocyte transformation and the animals were bled for serum to test for antibody production. Control mice were inoculated with tissue culture fluid. The transformation response of lymph node cells to Sindbis virus was shown to be specific and dependent on the amount of viral antigen used for stimulation. Sindbis virus does not infect lymphocytes or macrophages. Both live virus and virus inactivated by exposure to ultraviolet light were used as antigen (Table 1). Live virus was

Table 1

Dose Response of Sindbis Virus-Sensitized Lymph Node Cells

to Live and UV-Inactivated Sindbis Virus Antigen

Dilution	Live			UV-Inactivated	
	pfu	cpm	LT index	cpm	LT index
10^0	$10^{7.1}$	16538	53	---	---
$10^{-.5}$	$10^{6.6}$	11030	35.5	646	2.1
10^{-1}	$10^{6.1}$	3811	12.3	367	1.2
10^{-2}	$10^{5.1}$	610	2.0	414	1.3

(From Griffin and Johnson, 1973)

Reprinted with permission from Academic Press.

a much more effective antigen for lymphocyte transformation than was inactivated virus. Perhaps it makes more effective contact with a sensitized lymphocyte by attaching and perhaps penetrating the cells without being able to damage the cell by replicating within it.

The time needed to develop sensitized lymph node cells is shown in Fig. 4. Sensitized cells were detectable in draining lymph nodes 3-4 days after infection. The cellular response increased rapidly with a peak at 6-7 days and then diminished rapidly to undetectable levels by day 15. Spleen cells showed a more gradual response which was much less

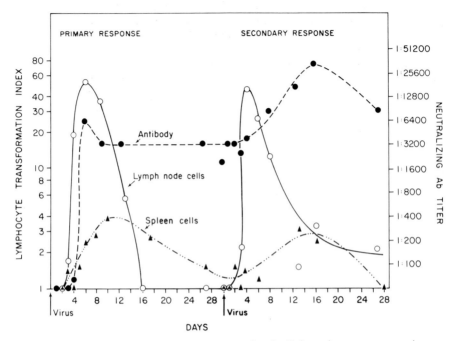

Fig. 4. Temporal development of Sindbis virus-responsive cells in the draining lymph nodes and spleen, and of neutralizing antibody after subcutaneous inoculation of Sindbis virus. (from Griffin and Johnson, 1973). Reprinted with permission from Academic Press.

pronounced than that in the draining lymph node. If the immune mouse was given a second inoculum of Sindbis virus (either live or inactivated) at 30 days it generated an anamnestic response peaking at day 4-5. In contrast to the evanescent cellular immune response to Sindbis virus as measured by lymphocyte transformation, the neutralizing antibody response remained elevated at 30 days and was boosted somewhat by rechallenge.

T AND B CELL COOPERATION

Whether the sensitized lymphocytes stimulated in vitro by Sindbis virus are T cells or B cells is a question which can be answered in the mouse. Theta (θ) antigen is a surface marker which precursor cells acquire when they are processed by the thymus to become functional T cells (21). Easily detectable immunoglobulin is present on the surface of B cells

(21). Therefore T and B cells can be evaluated separately by pretreating the mixed population with either anti- θ or anti-mouse immunoglobulin antisera plus complement to selectively destroy one cell population. When either T cells or B cells are tested in this way for a specific response to Sindbis virus most of the reactivity is in the T cell population, but B cells do contribute somewhat to the response (Table 2). A contribution from both cell populations is not

Table 2

The Effect of Pretreating Sindbis Virus-Sensitized Cells with

Serum and Complement on the Stimulation of ^{3}H-Tdr Incorporation

by PHA and Sindbis Virus Antigen[a]

Treatment	cpm control	cpm PHA	LT index	cpm control	cpm Sindbis	LT index
Normal mouse serum	229	12616	55	342	1598	4.7
Anti-θ serum	240	768	3.2	326	361	1.1
Normal rabbit serum	211	24227	114	328	2687	8.2
Anti-Mouse Immuno-globulin	310	12209	39	278	983	3.5

[a]Average of 3 experiments   Reprinted with permission from
(From Griffin and Johnson, 1973)   Academic Press, Inc.

surprising since there is evidence in infected animals of both a cell-mediated immune response (T cells) in the form of the mononuclear inflammation at sites of virus replication and a humoral immune response (B cells) in the form of high titers of virus neutralizing antibody.

The development of virus-specific cytotoxic lymphocytes in Sindbis virus-infected mice has also been studied (22). Sindbis virus-immune lymph node cells were capable of lysing acutely infected mouse embryo fibroblasts bearing surface viral antigen before viral-induced lysis occurred. The effector cell in this in vitro assay was a T cell, and the cytotoxic reaction could be blocked by Sindbis virus-immune serum.

The most difficult question to be answered is what role the immune responses, both cellular and humoral, have in recovery from the disease. The fact that cyclophosphamide immunosuppression delays viral clearance suggests that immunologic processes may be responsible for clearance of virus from the brain. Brain virus was quantitated 3-4 days after transfer of immune serum or cells into Sindbis virus-infected immunosuppressed mice (14). Immune serum decreased the titer a hundred-fold from $10^{5.7}$ to $10^{3.8}$ plaque forming units (pfu)/gram brain and the immune lymph node cells decreased virus content a thousand-fold from $10^{5.7}$ to $10^{2.7}$ pfu/gram brain. In vitro studies have shown (22) that viral clearance in the absence of antibody is dependent on a population of noncytotoxic, adherent cells, probably macrophages. These data suggest that recovery depends on a balance between lymphocyte-mediated lysis of infected cells and viral clearance by macrophages and antibody.

An additional approach to the question of the role of the immune response in recovery from Sindbis virus encephalitis has been to develop a strain of Sindbis virus which kills weanling mice instead of causing a nonfatal infection. In order to produce such a strain Sindbis virus was passed by intracerebral inoculation into suckling mice. After the sixth passage this Sindbis virus (MP6) reproducibly killed weanling mice at 6-10 days after intracerebral inoculation. Studies were then done to ascertain what role immune cells or serum passively transferred into these non-immunosuppressed mice would have on the outcome of the fatal infection. Preliminary studies with this strain indicate that mice can be protected if immune serum or cells are passively transferred 24 hours after intracerebral inoculation with 10 50% intracerebral lethal doses (IC LD_{50}) of MP6 virus. Immune serum appears to protect better and later than either immune spleen cells or immune lymph node cells. The mechanism of this protection is a subject of current investigations, but does not appear to be related to direct neutralization of infectious Sindbis virus (Griffin, unpublished data).

In summary, a detailed study of Sindbis virus infection in the mouse has elucidated a number of basic parameters of the interaction between virus and host. Sindbis virus encephalitis involves a rapid growth of this lytic arbovirus in cells of the central nervous system. In the weanling mouse neutralizing antibody and sensitized lymphoid cells are detectable between 3-4 days after infection and at this time a virus-specific perivascular mononuclear inflammation appears. Clearance of the virus from the brain occurs between day 6-7 at a time when antibody titers and the cell mediated immune response of lymph node cells to Sindbis virus antigen reach a peak. Neutralizing antibody remains high while detectable sensitized lymphoid cells decrease rapidly. The relative importance of immune cells and immune serum in recovery have not yet been clearly delineated but both appear to be important.

This investigation was supported by the Benjamin Miller Grant for Research on Multiple Sclerosis from the National Multiple Sclerosis Society (628-B-5) and Public Health Service Grant 5-P01-NS10920-2 from the National Institute of Neurological Diseases and Stroke, National Institutes of Health.

REFERENCES

1. Fenner, F. (1968). The Biology of Animal Viruses. Vol. I. Molecular and Cellular Biology. Academic Press, New York.
2. Fenner, F. (1968). The Biology of Animal Viruses. Vol. II. The pathogenesis and ecology of viral infections. Academic Press, New York.
3. Johnson, R.T. (1970). J. Infect. Dis. 121: 227.
4. Bloom, B.R. (1969). In Mediators of Cellular Immunity (Lawrence,H.S. and Landy, M., ed.) p. 247. Academic Press, New York.
5. Oldstone, M.B.A., and Dixon, F.J.(1970) J. Immunol.105:829.
6. Notkins, A.L. (1971). J. Exp. Med. 134: 41s.
7. Notkins, A.L., Mergenhagen, S.E. and Howard, R.J. (1970). Ann. Rev. Microbiol. 24: 525.
8. Malherbe, H., Strickland-Cholmley, M., and Jackson, A.L. (1963). S. Afr. Med. J. 37: 547.
9. Johnson, R.T. (1965). American J. Pathol. 46: 929.
10. Johnson, R.T., McFarland, H.F. and Levy, S.E. (1972). J. Infect. Dis. 125: 257.
11. Johnson, R.T. (1969). Res. Publ. Assoc. Res. Nerv. Ment. Dis. 49: 305.
12. Rivers, T.M. (1928). American J. Pathol. 4: 91.
13. Buddingh, G.J. (1965). In Viral and Rickettsial Infections of Man (Horsfall, F.L. and Tamm, I.,ed.) p. 339. J.B. Lippincott Co., Philadelphia 4th ed.
14. McFarland, H.F., Griffin, D.E. and Johnson, R.T.(1972). J. Exp. Med. 136: 216.

15. Bloom, B.R. and Glade, P.R. (1971). In Vitro Methods in Cell-mediated Immunity. Academic Press, New York.
16. Janossy, G. and Greaves, M.F. (1971). Clin. Exp. Immunol. 9: 483.
17. Moller, G. Sjoberg, O. and Andersson, J. (1973). J. Infect. Dis. 128: supplement: 552.
18. Stockman, G.D., Gallagher, M.T., Heim, L.R., South, M.A. and Trentin, J.J. (1971). Proc. Soc. Exp. Biol. Med. 136: 980.
19. Benezra, D., Gery,I.and Davies, A.M. (1969). Clin. Exp. Immunol. 5: 155
20. Griffin, D.E. and Johnson, R.T. (1973). Cell. Immunol. 9: 426.
21. Raff, M.C. (1970). Immunol. 19: 637.
22. McFarland, H.F. (1974). J. Immunol. 113: 173.

6

Viral-Induced Immunopathology
Donald H. Gilden

Immune responsiveness and disease (pathology) may occur simultaneously. Immunopathology can be viewed as immune phenomena and reactions associated with injury to the host. Since many viruses are potent antigens (1), it follows that host immune responsiveness to viral infection might occasionally be associated with viral-induced immunopathology. More definitive information is needed relating the role of immune reactions to the pathogenesis of viral infection in man. However, experimental models of viral-induced immunopathology exist, the prototype being the unique relationship between lymphocytic choriomeningitis (LCM) virus and the mouse.

LCM virus belongs to the arenavirus group, a recently proposed name based on the granular appearance of virus particles (Arenosus--sandy) by electron microscopy (2). The arenaviruses contain RNA (3,4,5), are lipid solvent sensitive (6), and some share a common immunofluorescent and complement-fixing antigen (7). Virus particles are pleomorphic, varying in size from 50-300 nanometers, and they are released from infected cells by budding (8). The arenavirus group consists of Amapari, Junin, Lassa, Latino, LCM (the prototype), Machupo, Parana, Pichinde, Tacaribe, and Tamiami viruses.

Immunopathology has been clearly demonstrated not only secondary to LCM infection but also following inoculation of other arenaviruses into susceptible rodents [Junin (9),

DONALD H. GILDEN

Tacaribe (10), and Tamiami (11)]. However, the mechanisms
of viral-induced immune mediated disease have been far more
extensively investigated with LCM virus; thus only the dis-
section of the LCM virus-mouse relationship is germane to
this chapter.

Numerous pathogenesis studies of central nervous system
(CNS) virus infection revealed decreased host susceptibility
with increasing age (12,13). Yet intracerebral (IC) inoculation of the adult mouse with LCM virus is regularly followed
by death within 6-7 days while IC inoculation of the newborn
mouse immediately after birth fails to produce acute neurologic disease and results in a persistently infected carrier.
The exact reversal of the expected increased susceptibility
of the newborn to withstand IC virus challenge led Burnet to
postulate that virus introduction during a stage of relative
immunologic immaturity resulted in the virus being recognized
as "self" while acute neurologic disease which followed IC
inoculation of virus in the adult resulted from an immunocompetent hose response (14).

In vitro studies demonstrating that mouse fibroblast cell
lines were not altered or destroyed by LCM virus while con-
tinuing to produce considerable amounts of infectious virus
(15) provided more presumptive evidence that pathology from
LCM virus might not be due to virus alone.

Further substantiation that immune responsiveness played
a role in the outcome following LCM virus infection was provided by the beneficial effect of immunosuppression. A potentially lethal infection could be converted into a chronic
carrier state, despite high titers of virus in brain and
other tissues. Various immunosuppressive techniques were ex-
ploited including X-irradiation (16,17), anti-lymphocyte se-
rum(18),neonatal thymectomy(19) and Cyclophosphamide(CY) (20).

The Cyclophosphamide model of immunosuppression provided
a technique to study the dynamic relationship between virus
replication and immune response. Weanling BALB/c mice inoculated IC with Armstrong strain of LCM virus developed acute
neurologic disease 6-7 days later which was corroborated by
acute meningitis (Fig. 1a) and choroiditis (Fig. 1b).
Immunofluorescent studies demonstrated LCM viral antigen confined to the choroid plexus, ependyma, and meninges (Fig. 2).
Weanling BALB/c mice inoculated with LCM virus and given
Cyclophosphamide 150 mgms./kg. intraperitoneally (IP) 3 days
after infection were spared from acute neurologic disease.
If sacrificed at parallel times when clinical and histologi-
cal disease was manifest in the non-immunosuppressed mouse,
the meninges, ependyma, and choroid plexus appeared normal
(Fig. 3), yet immunofluorescent examination revealed an

84

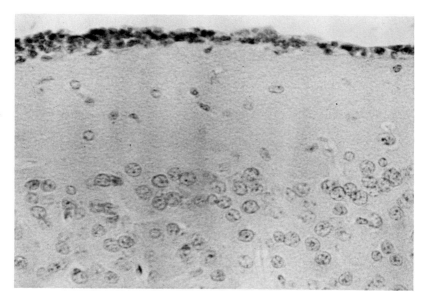

Fig. 1(a) Meninges and underlying cerebral cortex from an adult mouse inoculated IC with LCM virus and perfused when moribund 6 days later. Hematoxylin and erythrosin. X128.

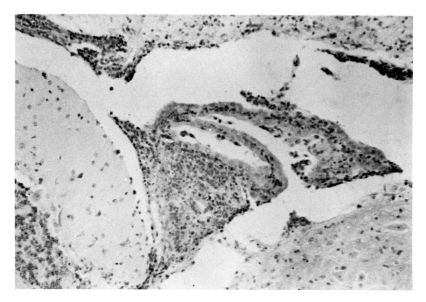

Fig. 1(b) Choroid plexus of fourth ventricle from adult mouse inoculated IC with LCM virus and perfused when moribund 7 days later. Hematoxylin and erythrosin. X150.

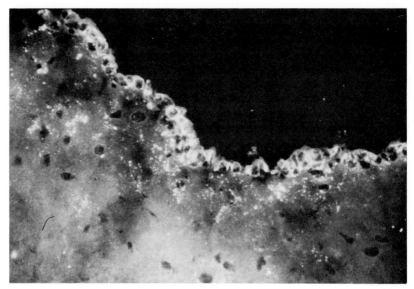

Fig. 2. Infection of leptomeninges of cerebral cortex from an adult mouse inoculated IC with LCM virus, given CY (150 mg/kg) 3 days later and asymptomatic when perfused 7 days after virus infection. Anti-LCM immunofluorescent stain. X175.

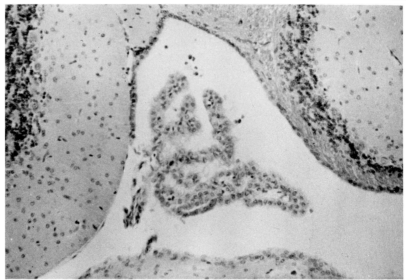

Fig. 3. Choroid plexus of fourth ventricle from an adult mouse inoculated IC with LCM virus, given CY (150 mg/kg) 3 days later, and asymptomatic when perfused 16 days after virus infection. Hematoxylin and erythrosin. X150.

identical distribution of viral antigen in the choroid plexus, ependyma, and meninges. Brains from both LCM-inoculated moribund mice and from asymptomatic LCM virus-infected Cyclophosphamide (drug) immunosuppressed mice were also titered for the presence of virus on day 7 and found to contain equivalent amounts of virus particles. The single dose of Cyclophosphamide 3 days after IC inoculation of LCM virus converted more than 80% of mice into LCM carriers, clinically identical to neonatally infected carrier mice.

In summary: IC inoculation of LCM virus produces acute choriomeningitis in weanling or adult mice in 7 days. Cyclophosphamide protects these mice from acute CNS disease despite equal concentration and distribution of virus in CNS target tissue (choroid plexus, meninges, and ependyma) 7 days after infection: the time when non-immunosuppressed mice are dying.

Unequivocal evidence that immune mechanisms play a role in disease production comes from adoptive immunization (transfer) studies. In this procedure immunocytes from animals challenged with antigen (here: LCM virus) are passively transferred to recipients in an attempt to produce disease. These experimental techniques were originally problematic presumably because transferred cells were rejected by outbred animals. However, this problem has been surmounted by using inbred isogenic mouse strains.

Original attempts to produce acute LCM disease by adoptive immunization were carried out using neonatally infected carrier mice as recipients (21). Lymphoid tissue from LCM-immune BALB/c mice effectively terminated tolerance reducing virus levels in the blood by 3 logs while antibody production reached very high levels. However clinical disease did not develop. Reasons for the failure of adoptive transfer to produce disease in these recipients include the following:

First, there is a difference between the distribution of viral antigen in the brain. Only a few viral antigen containing cells are seen in the choroid plexus and meninges of neonatally induced carriers. The choroid plexus and meninges of drug induced carriers, however, are heavily laden with LCM viral antigen indicating that these cells are better targets for the antiviral immune response than the same tissue in the neonatally induced carrier (22).

Second, is the greater tissue and blood concentration of virus in the neonatally induced carrier in contrast to the drug induced carrier. Binding of immunocompetent cells by viral antigen prior to the entrance of cells into the CNS may account for the lack of disease in the neonatally induced carrier (22). One can see a similar phenomenon in experimental allergic encephalomyelitis (EAE) if basic protein is administered prior to adoptive immunization. This prevents the development of neurological disease (cited in 22).

Further experiments to produce acute lymphocytic chorio-meningitis by adoptive immunization were performed in the following manner: Recipients were Cyclophosphamide induced LCM carrier BALB/c mice. Donor cells came from adult BALB/c mice that had been given repeated inoculations of the Arm-strong strain of LCM virus intraperitoneally (IP) which results in a non-fatal immunizing infection (23). The series of inoculations were carried out over a 6-8 week period, the last "booster" given 7-10 days before adoptive transfer. The procedure for removal and preparation of immune and control spleen cells and serum from donors has been described (22). Donor cells were administered IP and serum was given intravenously (IV).

Table 1 demonstrates the ability of immune spleen cells from hyperimmunized mice to produce acute lymphocytic chorio-meningitis in "destined-to-survive" Cyclophosphamide induced carrier mice. These same carrier mice given normal spleen cells or immune serum failed to develop disease. Clinical disease developed 6-8 days after cell transfer and was characterized by hunched posture, ruffled fur, tremulousness and little body movements. Often a convulsion heralded the onset of death. These typical features of acute lymphocytic choriomeningitis were confirmed histopathologically by an intense choriomeningitis (Fig. 4).

The LCM model described above provides an opportunity to analyze the mechanisms of viral-induced immunopathology. What is the role, for example, of donor vs. recipient contribution to immunopathology? The fact that 6-8 days are required before disease ensues after adoptive transfer suggests that donor spleen cells do not react directly with infected central nervous system tissue. Recipient participation in other systems has been suggested by studies of a different, non-viral, immune mediated disease of the CNS, experimental allergic encephalomyelitis. In this disorder, 4-8 days are also needed for adoptive transfer to produce disease. Equally interesting is the failure of adoptive transfer to produce EAE in the neonatal rat due to presumed immunologic immaturity of the recipient (24). Mechanisms operable in EAE may also occur in the production of viral-induced immuno-pathology.

Another issue is that of humoral vs. cellular factors in producing acute LCM disease. If cells are responsible, are they T, B, or both? Using the experimental model previously described, Cole has demonstrated that treatment of the

CONVERSION OF LCM VIRUS CARRIER STATES TO LETHAL

CHORIOMENINGITIS FOLLOWING TRANSFER OF IMMUNE

SYNGENEIC SPLEEN CELLS

LCM Virus 1000 LD50 Day 0	Cyclophosphamide 150 mg/k Day 3	Spleen Cells ($\pm 10^8$)	Dead/Total*	Per cent Mortality
+	-	-	40/40	100
+	+	-	5/110	0-10
-	+	-	2/50	0-5
+	+	Immune		
		Day 5	32/32	100
		Day 25	28/29	97
		Day 40	34/34	100
		Day 330	6/6	100
+	+	Normal		
		Day 5	5/20	25
		Day 25	0/24	0

immune spleen cells with anti-theta serum rendered donor cells incapable of producing acute LCM disease in drug-induced carrier mice, but did not eliminate their ability to produce antibody (25). Furthermore, Cole and coworkers demonstrated presumptive evidence of virus-antibody complexes in the brain. Immunofluorescent staining revealed both viral antigen and immunoglobulin at identical sites within the central nervous system in asymptomatic mice adoptively immunized with anti-theta serum-treated spleen cells. These clinically well mice continued to produce antibody. One can postulate that theta-bearing lymphocytes are required for the production of acute lymphocytic choriomeningitis, and that the presence of both LCM specific viral antigen and immunoglobulin in identical CNS sites of asymptomatic mice argue against the role of immune complexes in mediating acute CNS disease.

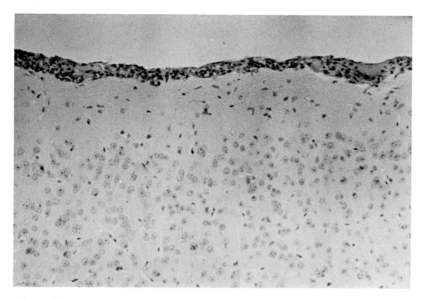

Fig. 4. Severe leptomeningitis in an adult mouse inoculated IC with LCM virus (day 0), treated with CY on day 3, adoptively immunized with isogenic spleen cells from an immunized donor on day 5, and perfused when moribund on day 10. Hematoxylin and erythrosin. X150.

Further studies indicating that T cells play a role in the production of acute LCM disease are provided by Zinkernagel (26) who demonstrated that thymus derived lymphocytes which are cycotoxic for LCM-infected L cells have been found in the spleens of mice 6 days after infection with LCM virus and are increased the next day when all mice are clinically ill. Not only did symptomatology parallel the development of cytotoxic cells in lymphoid tissue, but cytotoxic T cells were also demonstrated in the cerebral spinal fluid at the same time (26).

A final point of conjecture is how virus might cause immunopathology. Most of the presumed mechanisms (Table 2) operable in viral-induced immunopathology are provoked by either the virion or its subcomponents which may be presented as the neoantigen. Its release from infected cells may provoke a non-beneficial immune response. Neoantigen on the surface of infected cells may also stimulate effector T lymphocytes producing tissue destruction. Another means by which viruses may produce immunopathology involves immune complexes. Deposition of viral antigen, specific antibody, and complement may lead to cell death. Proof that immune com-

TABLE 2

POSSIBLE MECHANISMS OF VIRAL-INDUCED IMMUNOPATHOLOGY

A. VIRUS OR VIRUS-SPECIFIED NEOANTIGEN

1. Virus or subvirion components or virus-specified non-
    structural protein equals neoantigen.

2. Neoantigen is released from infected cells and calls
    forth an immune response.

3. Free neoantigen plus antibody form an immune complex
    which binds complement and leads to immune complex
    disease.

4. Neoantigen on the surface of infected cells plus
    antibody plus complement may lead to cell death
    (+ lysis).

5. Neoantigen on the surface of infected cells may
    stimulate effector T lymphocytes leading to cell death.

6. Neoantigen on the surface of infected cells plus
    normal antibody (cytophilic antibody) plus normal
    (non-sensitized) lymphocytes may lead to cell death
    (so-called antibody-dependent lymphocytolysis).

B. HOST-SPECIFIED ANTIGEN

1. Virus may alter host cells (normally non-immunogenic)
    so that they are rendered antigenic (so-called auto-
    immunity).

plexes produce acute LCM disease is wanting, although there
is evidence that immune complexes may play a role in the
renal disease which develops in LCM carrier mice (27).

A further method by which viruses may induce immunopathology is that of antibody-dependent lymphocytolysis. Neoantigen
on the surface of infected cells combined with normal (cyto-
philic) antibody may, in the presence of non-sensitized lymphocytes, produce cell death. This system does not involve
binding of complement. Although the relationship of antibody-dependent lymphocytolysis to viral-induced immunopathology in vivo is still theoretical, immunological destruction

of herpes simplex virus infected cells by antibody and non-immune effector cells (macrophages) in vitro has been demonstrated (28). One other postulated mechanism by which viruses may induce immunopathology is that virus may alter host cells so that they are rendered antigenic triggering an auto-immune response (29).

Whether any of these mechanisms play a role in the production of acute LCM disease is uncertain. However, in vitro correlates of LCM virus-induced immune responses have shown that the susceptibility of target cells to immune-mediated lysis by T-lymphocytes correlated with the density of immuno-fluorescent virus antigen on the cell surface (30). Yet cell lysis by antibody and complement seemed indèpendent of target cell density surface virus antigen. Furthermore, skin grafts from LCM carrier mice are rejected by uninfected syngeneic recipients (31). The above studies suggest that virus specific surface antigens may play a role in disease production.

Evidence so far indicates that cell mediated immunopathology against LCM virus operates both in vivo and in vitro. T lymphocytes react with LCM specific viral antigen to produce acute LCM disease. Further complicating adoptive immunization studies is recent evidence that fatal LCM disease depends upon sharing, by donor and recipient, of at least 1 set of H-2 antigenic specificities (32). Whether this presumed histocompatibility antigen may act as a receptor for a particular virus on the cell surface or may cross-react with a major antigenic determinant on a virus protein coat and lead to tolerance of the invading virus is not known (33). Finally, others have been unable to confirm the claim that acute LCM disease in the mouse is controlled by a gene closely linked to the H-2 locus (34).

Why immunopathology occurs only in the choroid plexus, meninges, ependyma, and under certain circumstances in cerebellar granule cells and white matter while sparing so many other parenchymal sites bearing LCM viral antigen is uncertain. These and other questions previously raised provide an impetus for further studies on the mechanisms of viral-induced immunopathology.

This work was supported in part by Public Health Service Research Grant NS11036 and NS09779 from the National Institute of Neurological Diseases & Stroke, National Institutes of Health and Grant RR05540 from the Division of Research Resources, The John A. Hartford Foundation, Inc., and a Grant from the National Multiple Sclerosis Society.

REFERENCES

1. Thorbecke, G.J. and Benacerraf, B. (1962). Progress in Allergy 6: 559.
2. Murphy, F.A., Webb, P.A., Johnson, K.M. and Whitfield, S. G. (1969). J. Virol. 4: 535.
3. Pfau, C.J. (1965). Acta Pathol. Microbiol.,Scandinavia,, 63: 188.
4. Pfau, C.J. (1965). Acta Pathol. Microbiol., Scandinavia, 63: 198.
5. Barlow, J.L. and Keller, E. (1965). In: Annual Report, New York State Dept. of Health (Albany), Div. of Laboratories and Research, p. 51.
6. Stock, C.C. and Francis, T., Jr. (1943). J. Exp. Med. 77: 323.
7. Rowe, W.P., Murphy, F.A.,Bergold, G.H., Casals, J., et.al. (1970). J. Virol. 5: 651.
8. Dalton, A.J., Rowe, W.P., Smith, G.H., et.al. (1968). J. Virol. 2: 1465.
9. Weissenbacher, M.C., Schmunis, G.A. and Parodi, A.S.(1969). Arch. Ges. Virusforsch. 26: 63.
10. Borden, E.C., Murphy, F.A., Nathanson, N. and Monath, T. P.C. (1971). Infect. Immun. 3: 466.
11. Gilden, D.H., Friedman, H.N., Kyj, C.O., et.al. (1973). In: Lymphocytic Choriomeningitis Virus and Other Arenaviruses. (Lehmann-Grube, F., ed.), p. 287, Springer-Verlag, New York.
12. Lennette, E.H. and Koprowski, H. (1944). J. Immunol. 49: 175.
13. Schlesinger, R.W. and Frankel, J.W. (1952). Am. J. Trop. Med. 1: 66.
14. Burnet, F.M. and Fenner, F. (1949). The Production of Antibodies, 2nd Edition, McMillan Co., Melbourne.
15. Lehmann-Grube, F. (1967). Nature (London) 213: 770.
16. Rowe, W.P. (1954). Res. Rep. Nav. Med. Res. Inst. 12:167.
17. Hotchin, J. and Weigand, H. (1961). J. Immunol. 86: 392.
18. Hirsch, M.S., Murphy, F.A. and Hicklin, M.D. (1968). J. Exp. Med., 127: 757.
19. Rowe, W.P., Black, P.H. and Levy, R.H. (1963). Proc. Soc. Exp. Biol. Med. 114: 248.
20. Gilden, D.H., Cole, G.A., Monjan, A.A. and Nathanson, N. (1972). J. Exp. Med. 135: 860.
21. Volkert, M. and Hannover Larsen, J. (1964). Acta Pathol. Microbiol., Scand. 60: 577.
22. Gilden, D.H., Cole, G.A. and Nathanson, N. (1972). J. Exp. Med. 135: 874.

23. Cole, G.A., Gilden, D.H., Monjan, A.A. and Nathanson, N. (1971). Fed. Proc. 30: 1831.
24. Paterson, P.Y. (1960). J. Exp. Med. 111: 119.
25. Cole, G.A., Nathanson, N. and Prendergast, R.A. (1972). Nature (London) 238: 335.
26. Zinkernagel, R.M. and Doherty, P.C. (1973). J. Exp. Med. 138: 1266.
27. Oldstone, M.B.A. and Dixon, F.J. (1971). J. Exp. Med. 134: 32s.
28. Rager-Zisman, B. and Bloom, B.R. (1974). Nature 251: 542.
29. Miescher, F.A. and Muller-Eberhard, J.H. (1968-1969). Textbook of Immunopathology, Vols. I & II. Grune and Stratton, New York.
30. Cole, G.A., Prendergast, R.A. and Henney, C.S. (1972). In: Lymphocytic Choriomeningitis Virus and Other Arenaviruses. (Lehmann-Grube, F., ed.) p. 61, Springer-Verlag, New York.
31. Holtermann, O.A. and Majde, J.A. (1971). Transplantation 11: 20.
32. Zinkernagel, R.M. and Doherty, P.C. (1974). Nature 248: 701.
33. McDevitt, H.O., Oldstone, M.B.A., and Pincus, T. (1974). Transplant. Rev. 19: 209.
34. Lehmann-Grube, F. (1969). Arch. Virusforsch. 28: 303.

7

Immune Complexes and Autoimmune Disease

Alfred D. Steinberg

INTRODUCTION

In this chapter we will illustrate "autoimmunity" with the
spontaneously occurring disease of New Zealand mice. In
these animals genetic and viral factors appear to influence
the immune system to produce an immune complex disease which
is complicated and yet understandable in terms of fundamental
principles.

First, is a summary of some of the features of disease in
New Zealand mice and humans with a related disorder, systemic
lupus erythematosus (SLE). We then progress from what is
known about immune complexes in specific viral infections to
the immune complexes in New Zealand mice and patients with
SLE. Next·, the concept of suppressor cells as illustrated by
immune enhancement with injections of anti-lymphocyte serum
is discussed. Finally, the subject of spontaneously occurring anti-thymocyte antibody in New Zealand mice which may
have profound effects on the immune system is presented,
leading into a closing discussion of the regulation of the
immune system and the role of its derangement in the pathogenesis of autoimmunity in New Zealand mice.

New Zealand mice and humans with SLE develop autoimmune
diseases which include multiple autoantibodies and immune
complex renal disease. The disease in New Zealand black(NZB)

mice is characterized by Coombs' positive hemolytic anemia,
lymphoid infiltration of many organs and membranous glomerulonephritis. When NZB mice are mated to New Zealand white
mice the offspring (NZB/NZW) have more severe glomerulonephritis and less prominent Coombs' positive hemolytic anemia.
Antibodies to nucleic acids are found in greater quantities
in NZB/NZW mice whereas anti-thymocyte antibodies are found
earlier and in higher titers in NZB mice. The cause(s) of
autoimmune disease in human systemic lupus and New Zealand
mice is unknown; however, evidence has accumulated which im-
plicates genetic, immunologic and viral factors.

   Antibodies to double stranded DNA which occur in high titer only in patients with SLE and in New Zealand mice are
thought to be characteristic of these diseases. Figure I
illustrates the increase with age in antibodies to DNA meas-

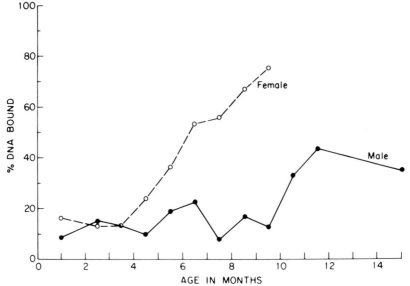

Fig. 1. Age and sex dependent formation of anti-DNA antibodies in NZB/NZW mice. Reprinted with permission from the
Williams and Wilkins Co., Maryland. (1).

ured by a modification of the Farr assay (1). Females develop
large quantities of anti-DNA much earlier in life than do
males. Castration and treatment with opposite sex hormones
does not turn a male anti-DNA pattern into a female pattern
or vice versa (2). These studies suggest that a gene exists
on the X chromosomes which is associated with the production
of antibodies to DNA. Such a gene was suggested by the
greater antibody response of female mice, over their geneti-

cally identical brothers, and to injection with synthetic double
stranded RNA antigens in aqueous solution as shown in Table
I (2). Recent genetic studies have demonstrated such an

TABLE I*

IMMUNIZATION OF NZB/NZW MICE

WITH MULTIPLE INJECTIONS OF rI·rC AND rA·rU

Injection	Antibody to rI·rC (μg./ml.)	
	Male	Female
rA·rU	1.6	7.6
rI·rC	3.9	15.9
Controls	0.8	1.6

*see ref. (2).

X-linked immune response gene in the antibody response to a
synthetic double stranded RNA, polyinosinic·polycytidylic
acid (rI·rC) (3). As a result of the more regular development of disease in female NZB/NZW mice, many studies have
been confined to females.

The natural history of NZB/NZW female mice consists of a
period of about three months during which time they are clinically well although a number of immunological abnormalities
may be demonstrated. Between three and six months of age
serum antibodies to nucleic acids become more and more easily
demonstrated as do renal deposits of immunoglobulin and complement. The complexes are first deposited in the mesangial
regions and later along the glomerular capillary walls.
Fluorescent microscopy using fluorescein conjugated antisera
to mouse antibody or complement components demonstrates deposition in a finely granular pattern followed by a coarsely
granular or "lumpy bumpy" pattern corresponding to areas of
electron dense deposits observed by electron microscopy.
Thereafter, histologically evident glomerulonephritis is followed by proteinuria a few months later and death from uremia
about one month after the onset of heavy proteinuria.

NZB/NZW mice develop, in addition to antibodies to DNA,
antibodies to double stranded RNA (4). The age associated
formation of these antibodies is illustrated in Figure II(2).
Since there is little double stranded RNA in mammalian

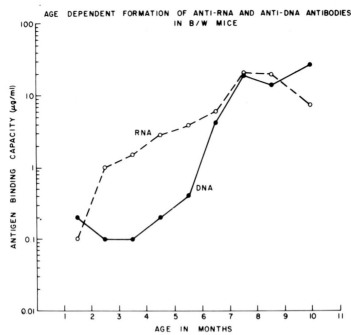

Fig. II. Age dependent formation of antibodies to double stranded RNA (o---o) and native DNA (●---●) in 16 NZB/NZW female mice bled serially for 10 months. Reprinted with permission from Blackwell Scientific Publications, England.[2].

---

tissues, it is possible that these antibodies are produced in response to viral double stranded RNA. It was of interest to find that patients with SLE also develop spontaneously antibodies to double stranded RNA (4). The prevalence of antibodies to double stranded RNA is illustrated in Table II (5). Such antibodies appear to have greater reactivity with viral than synthetic double stranded polyribonucleotides (6) as illustrated in Table III. It is also apparent that there is greater specificity for double stranded RNA than single stranded RNA. The naturally occurring antibodies resembled those induced by immunization with viral double stranded RNA to a greater extent than those induced by immunization with synthetic double stranded RNA (Table IV).

Multiple injections of rI·rC caused acceleration of disease in New Zealand mice (4,7) as shown in Figure III. Further study of mice first made tolerant to rI·rC (8) suggested that the RNA was acting both as an adjuvant and as an antigen (9). In these studies tolerant mice had accelerated anti-DNA production (adjuvant effect) without accelerated anti-RNA production (Figure IV). In another study we found that superinfection with Moloney leukemia virus (MLV) accelerated

98

TABLE II *
ANTIBODIES TO DOUBLE-STRANDED RNA
(POLY I·POLY C) IN HUMAN DISEASES

DISEASE STATE	NUMBER STUDIED	NUMBER POSITIVE	PERCENT POSITIVE
Normal	161	10	6
SLE	101	52	51
Pronestyl-SLE	25	3	12
RA	45	4	9
SS	28	2	7
Scleroderma	21	2	10
Myeloma	74	4	5

*see ref. (5).

Table III

COMPARATIVE ABILITY OF DIFFERENT RNAs TO INHIBIT
^{14}C rl · rC BINDING BY HUMAN LUPUS SERA

Serum	Percent Inhibition by							
	Reo	Phage	rl · rC	rA · rU	Ribosomal RNA Rat Liver	Transfer RNA Rat Liver	Transfer RNA E. coli	Transfer RNA Yeast
LN	100	100	86	81	42	32	32	25
IP	100	81	16	36	17	4	10	0
HR	100	62	77	36	54	21	37	23
BB	100	57	52	15	21	0	0	0
BD	91	51	21	42	7	0	0	0
AB	85	67	45	62	18	2	11	2
ML	74	62	23	93	35	3	17	2
GG	68	31	84	15	11	13	8	3
BA	47	59	25	30	19	3	0	8
Mean	85	63	47	45	24	8	12	7

Reprinted with permission from Rockefeller University Press, New York. (6).

TABLE IV

COMPARATIVE INHIBITION OF ANTIBODIES TO RNA

Antibody Source	No. of Sera	Percent of Sera giving I_{50} with			
		Rco	Phage	rI · rC	rA . rU
Human Lupus	18	72	50	55	39
Mouse Lupus	16	100	75	100	87
Immunized—phage	13	77	60	69	85
Immunized—rI · rC	12	17	12	100	83
Immunized—rA · rU	13	23	14	85	92

Reprinted with permission from Rockefeller University Press, New York. (6).

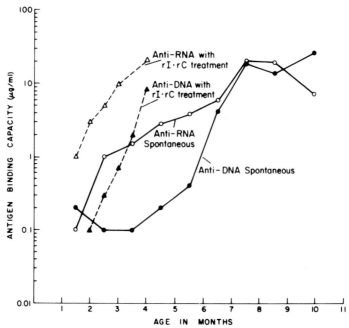

Fig.III. Accelerated formation of antibodies to double stranded RNA and native DNA induced by treatment of NZB/NZW female mice with rI.rC 100 μg. 3 X per week.
Reprinted with permission from Rockefeller Univ. Press, N.Y. (see ref. 10).

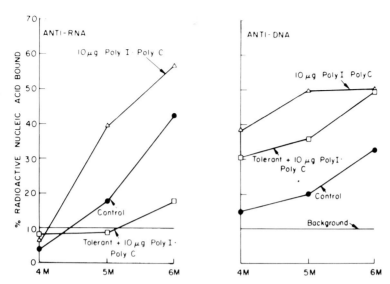

Fig. IV. Independent stimulation of antibodies to (a) double stranded RNA and (b) native DNA by poly I.poly C, 10 µg. 3X per week, after induction of tolerance in NZB, NZW females at 4 weeks of age. Reprinted with permission from Blackwell Scientific Publications, England. (9).

---

anti-RNA production of non-tolerant NZB/NZW mice (10). Induction of tolerance to RNA prevented this accelerated anti-RNA production by MLV.(Figure V).

Others have demonstrated accelerated disease following injection of DNA (11) and amelioration of disease following Statolon treatment (12) (See Wheelock, Chapter 4). Different viral infections can accelerate or retard disease in New Zealand mice. Studies suggest that the relationship between viral infection, nucleic acids and antinuclear antibodies in New Zealand mice is complex. It is further complicated by the presence in New Zealand mice of Gross virus which has been implicated as an important factor in the pathogenesis of their disease (13,14).

Drs. Oldstone and Dixon indicate that immune complex renal disease occurs frequently during the course of chronic viral infections in mice (15). Circulating immune complexes are demonstrated by the presence of virus-antibody-complement complexes in the circulation. These complexes appear to be deposited in the kidney where viral antigens, antibody and complement components are found by immunofluorescent techniques in a granular or "lumpy bumpy" pattern in the mesangium and later along glomerular capillary walls. Such immune

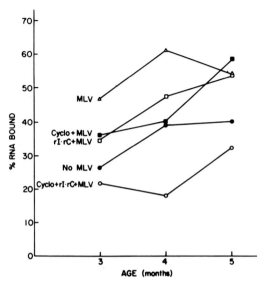

Fig. V.   Induction of tolerance to rI.rC prevents the
accelerated appearance of antibodies to RNA induced Moloney
leukemia virus in female NZB/NZW mice.   No MLV group control
mice.   Cyclo + rI.rC + MLV group = mice made tolerant to
rI.rC at 4 + 5 weeks of age and inoculated with MLV IP one
week later.   Cyclo + MLV group = control mice injected with
cyclophosphamide at 4 + 5 weeks of age and inoculated with
MLV one week later.   rI.rC + MLV group = control mice injected
with rI.rC at 4 + 5 weeks of age and inoculated with MLV one
week later.   Reprinted with permission from Federation of
American Societies for Experimental Biology, Maryland. (10).

complex disease has been found in mice chronically infected
with lymphocytic choriomeningitis virus (LCM), lactic dehydrogenase virus (LDV) and Moloney sarcoma virus.   Evidence
for immune complex deposits has also been found in Coxsackie
B, polyoma,Rauscher, Friend and Gross virus infections in
mice.   In Aleutian disease of mink antibody-virus immune complexes have been convincingly demonstrated.   Animals other
than rodents can be similarly affected as in equine anemia
and hog cholera.   These observations strongly suggest that
chronic viral illness may lead to immune complex disease and
chronic glomerulonephritis.   However, both the particular
agent and the genetic and immunologic state of the host appear to be important in determining whether or not clinically

significant renal disease will occur. Thus, SWR/J mice infected with LCM develop severe nephritis. The same strain
developed clinically insignificant immune complex disease
when infected with LDV. This was associated with a lesser
degree of immune complex deposition in the kidney suggesting
that secondary inflammatory factors were not the reason for
the difference. Furthermore, C3H mice infected with LCM did
not develop severe renal disease in contrast to the response
of SWR/J mice, suggesting a genetic component. This appeared
to be associated with a lesser degree of viremia in C3H mice
and fewer circulating complexes. A final important point to
emerge from this work was the finding that only half of the
antibody eluted from the kidney of mice infected with a
known virus was antibody which reacted with the infecting
virus. Therefore, additional immune complexes may occur during the course of chronic immune complex disease caused by a
known viral agent. The additional antibody appeared not to
be antinucleoprotein, and its specificity remains unknown.
A more recent paper by these authors has demonstrated that
large doses of cyclophosphamide given to chronic LCM carriers
could lead to the elimination of the host antibody response
(16). Although there was no change in the high viral titers
present in the serum, this reduction in the host immune response prevented the usual immune complex glomerulonephritis
(16). Similar results have been observed in Aleutian mink
disease (17). This is convincing evidence that the host antibody response to the viral agent is important in the production of disease. It also indicates that a favorable response
to an immunosuppressive drug does not mean that a disease is
not related to an infectious agent. The studies with LCM
also illustrate that an agent capable of producing an acute
fulminating disease in an adult may lead to a chronic illness
when contracted in utero or very early in life. The immature
immune system does not mount a strong immune response to
these viral antigens. As a result, viruses circulate in
large numbers and although antibody is made it is not enough
to eliminate the viremia. In fact, viruses circulate with
antibody and complement bound to their surfaces.

Since viruses are not eliminated from the circulation by
an adequate immune response but continue to circulate, the
host is susceptible to the deposition of virus-antibody complexes in the kidney, choroid plexus and other vessels over
a prolonged period of time. Eventually, the host's ability
to handle the deposition of these complexes is overcome and
clinical disease ensues. It is of interest that in the
presence of chronic viremia, free antiviral antibody does
not occur. It had been thought that this state represented

ALFRED D. STEINBERG

complete tolerance and that no antibody to virus was produced.
However, Dr. Notkins found that both antibody and complement
were present, attached to virus (18). Precipitation with
substances that bind either antibody or complement resulted
in lower virus titers in the remaining serum. Therefore,
the animals produce some antibody, but never enough to satu-
rate the large number of sites present on the viruses in the
circulation. These points are of particular relevance to
New Zealand mice, in which Gross virus is demonstrable in
utero. Unlike other strains, New Zealand mice lose their
tolerance to Gross viral antigens in a manner similar to
their loss of tolerance to self antigens.

Dixon, Oldstone and Tonietti examined the antibody eluted
from kidneys of New Zealand mice (19). Previous study by
Mellors and his colleagues had suggested that the naturally
occurring Gross virus infection of New Zealand mice induced
an antibody response leading to immune elimination of the
virus and deposition in the kidneys (13,14). I would like to
stress that in New Zealand mice no one has purposefully infected animals with virus. These mice naturally harbor Gross
virus as do many other strains. The other strains do not
develop autoimmunity suggesting that this host was unusual
(or perhaps that the virus was unusual).

Although Gross viral antigens and antibody had been demonstrated in the kidneys of New Zealand mice (14), the quantity
of antibody to Gross virus in the glomeruli was not known.
In addition, New Zealand mice and patients with SLE were
known to have antinuclear antibodies in their kidneys. Finally,
New Zealand mice make large antibody responses to a number of
self-antigens including nuclear and erythrocyte antigens.
Therefore, an attempt was made to elute antibody from the
kidneys of New Zealand mice and determine the quantity of
antibody reactive with Gross viral antigens and nuclear antigens.

The important contribution of Dr. Dixon and his collabora-
tors in this study was to go to a target organ and try to
elute the antibody deposited there, followed by an attempt at
quantifying the eluted antibody with regard to specificity.
Although these elution procedures have technical problems,
they represent a considerable advance over previous immunofluorescent studies. Using fluorescence microscopy, it is
not possible to tell whether the antibody to LCM in a kidney
represents 1% of all the antibody, 10%, or 95%. One can only
state that it is there. Being able to elute the antibody and
quantitate it allows one to appreciate the percentage of the
deposited antibodies having particular specificities. It was
found that considerably more antibodies to nuclear antigens

104

than to Gross antigens were found in the kidney eluates from NZB, NZW and NZB/NZW mice. Almost one-half of the antibody had specificity for nuclear antigens whereas 21% or less had specificity for Gross virus antigens. In contrast, SWR/J mice chronically infected with LCM and subjected to similar studies were found to have almost half of the eluted antibody reactive with LCM and only 3% with nuclear antigens.

We should pause for a moment to observe that the nucleoprotein antigen used in these studies might react with antibody that had specificity for double stranded DNA, single stranded DNA, histones, combinations of histones and either single or double stranded DNA, or other nuclear antigens. This should not detract from the study, but it is mentioned to indicate that a variety of antinuclear antibodies might be absorbed by nucleoprotein.

Superinfection of NZB, NZW and NZB/NZW mice with LCM and polyoma virus led to accelerated immune complex renal disease. Antibody eluted from such kidneys reacted with nuclear antigens (about 40% of the antibody) and the infecting virus (about 30% of the antibody). It was suggested that Gross virus infection of New Zealand mice was not unique in intensifying immune complex disease in New Zealand mice. Apparently, many viruses can induce immune complex disease in New Zealand mice which in combination with antinuclear antibody-antigen complexes leads to enhanced nephritis. However, not all viral infections of New Zealand mice which lead to antigen-antibody complexes also lead to increased nephritis. In contrast to the experiments with LCM and polyoma, superinfection of NZB/NZW mice with LDV leads to amelioration of disease, the mechanism of action being unclear (20). Taken together, these studies suggest that in a given spontaneously occurring immune complex disease, such as the autoimmune disease of New Zealand mice (or patients with SLE) more than one element may be acting simultaneously.

Genetic, immunologic and viral factors allow excessive antibody responses to viral, nuclear and other antigens which participate in the immune complex disease. These studies also suggest that only a very small percentage of all of the circulating complexes actually are deposited and remain in the kidney. Before going on, I would like to do a little arithmetic. Almost 50% of the antibody in the New Zealand mouse kidney reacts with nucleoproteins and 20% with Gross virus. Another 20% or so has been found to react with soluble erythrocyte antigens (21). It may soon be possible to account for the specificities of almost all of the antibody eluted from the kidneys of these animals.

Koffler, Agnello, Thoburn, and Kunkel showed that patients

with SLE may have high serum titers to many nuclear antigens
although there is no necessary correlation between the serum
antibody levels and antibody eluted from the patient's kidney (22). Antibodies to both native and denatured DNA were
found in the eluates of kidneys from patients with SLE. A
lesser incidence of antibodies to ribonucleoprotein was found.
Fluorescent studies suggested that rheumatoid factor might
also contribute to immune complex deposition either by fixing
to preformed complexes or as an independent γ globulin-anti-
γ globulin complex.

We will not discuss in detail the complex sequence of
events between deposition of antigen-antibody complexes and
clinical disease. They probably include activation of complement components leading to release of mediators and ulti-
mately an inflammatory response produced by leukocytes. It
might be worth mentioning that in addition to continued complex deposition other factors may act to perpetuate the inflammatory process. For example, sufficient renal inflammation could lead to release into the circulation of basement
membrane and tubular antigens. In certain instances these
might be immunogenic, leading to secondary causes of renal
disease even after immune complexes have ceased to be deposited.

There is, then, an indication that multiple immune complexes may be present in spontaneously occurring autoimmune
disease of mice and man. They further suggest that multiple
factors are involved in the pathogenesis of these disorders.
In order to study the role of immunologic factors we will
turn to the concept of regulatory function of the thymus in
the immune response and mechanisms whereby derangement of
such a regulatory role might lead to the excessive antibody
responses which would predispose to immune complex disease.

Type III pneumococcal polysaccharide (SSSIII) apparently
does not require helper T cells for the production of an
antibody response. Baker pointed out that administration of
an antiserum which inactivates mouse lymphocytes (ALS) at the
time of immunization with SSSIII leads to an enhanced antibody response to the SSSIII (23). This result suggested that
there were thymic derived regulatory or suppressor cells
which normally serve to inhibit or regulate the antibody response to SSSIII. In the absence of such regulatory cells,
the antibody response to SSSIII is enhanced. An alternative
explanation might be that the ALS acted as a non-specific
adjuvant. However, when thymocytes were given the next day
to animals who had received SSSIII plus ALS, a marked degree
of suppression of the antibody response to SSSIII was observed, suggesting that a non-specific adjuvant effect

was not responsible. Rather, it appeared that by restoring the suppressor cells killed by the ALS a response similar to that following SSSIII alone was observed. A second population of enhancing cells was found in the peripheral blood. These studies suggest that the cellular regulation of the antibody response to what had previously appeared to be a "thymic independent" antigen is in fact complicated. At least two populations of cells appear to regulate the response through enhancing or suppressing action.

Several early studies by Gershon and coworkers provided evidence for the existence of suppressor or regulatory cells for thymic-dependent responses (24). Additional studies of both thymic independent and thymic dependent immune responses have strengthened the concept of suppressor cells (25,26). The studies of Tada and coworkers strongly suggest antigen specific control of the IgE response to DNP-ascaris in the rat (27). Allotype suppression also seems to be associated with a suppressor T cell (28). Although numerous experiments have now demonstrated the phenomenon of suppression, a unique suppressor cell population has not yet been isolated and characterized.

Shirai and Mellors described an antibody to thymocytes which is produced spontaneously by New Zealand mice (29). Although some other mice produce such an antibody, New Zealand mice do so: 1) early in life; 2) uniformly and 3) in high titer as they age. This antibody reacts with thymocytes and is cycotoxic in vitro. It is possible that such an antibody could lead to the elimination of regulatory or suppressor cells. The spontaneous production of such an antibody in New Zealand mice might explain their excessive antibody responses to certain antigens such as nuclear antigens and viral antigens. Such an excessive antibody response might contribute to the immune complex renal disease observed in New Zealand mice. It remains to be determined to what extent such an antibody might lead to lymphoid cell death and release of nuclear antigens. Nuclear antigen release might result in immunization and later to combination with existing antinuclear antibodies.

I would like to conclude with some studies we have conducted which bear on the subject of loss of immunologic regulatory function in New Zealand mice. The first studies are based upon the antibody response to rI.rC which appears not to require many thymic helper cells (30,31). Figure VI illustrates that an injection of 100 μg rI.rC in aqueous solution leads to an antibody response in BALB/c mice with a peak at about 4 days (32). A second injection leads to a blunted response (Figure VI). Multiple injections lead to tolerance

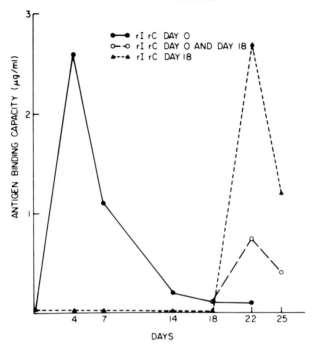

Fig. VI. Time course of tolerance to a second infection of rI.rC in BALB/c mice. Group of 12 mice was immunized with 100 μg. rI.rC on Day 0 and bled serially (●——●). On Day 18 6 of these mice were challenged with a second 100 μg. dose of rI.rC (o---o) and the remainder were not injected. Antibody response was determined at 4-7 days after secondary challenge. The response of a control group of mice simultaneously immunized for the first time on day 18 is shown (Δ_ _ _ Δ). Reprinted with permission from the Williams and Wilkins Co., Maryland. (32).

---

in BALB/c mice, but not in NZB/NZW mice (Table V). This is similar to impaired tolerance to serum protein antigens reported in New Zealand mice (33,34). It appeared that rather than hyper-responding to nucleic acid antigens, New Zealand mice had a more fundamental problem of impaired immunological regulation.

With the discovery that suppressor function could be studied by the administration of ALS as described above, we decided to study the response of NZB/NZW and control mice to rI.rC and anti-thymocyte serum (ATS) (31). The first study confirmed with rI.rC the observations made with SSSIII (Table VI). With age NZB/NZW mice lost the ability to have the anti-RNA response enhanced with ATS (Tables VII and VIII). These studies suggested an age associated loss of immune

TABLE V

ANTIBODY RESPONSE TO ONE OR MULTIPLE (3x/wk)
INJECTIONS OF rI·rC (100 μg) IN AQUEOUS SOLUTION

Strain	No.	ABC to rI·rC (μg/ml)	
		4 day	14 day
BALB/c	1	3.2	1.0
	12	0.7	< 0.5
NZB/W	1	3.6	0.8
	12	2.6	3.2

Reprinted with permission from the Williams and Wilkins Co.,
Maryland. (32).

TABLE VI

ENHANCED ANTIBODY RESPONSE OF BALB/c
MICE TO rI·rC (100μg) IN AQUEOUS SOLUTION
WHEN GIVEN WITH ATS

Treatment	ABC to rI·rC (μg/ml)	
	day 5	day 8
None	< 0.5	< 0.5
rI·rC	2.8	2.6
rI·rC + NRS	2.7	1.8
rI·rC + ATS	13.8	8.1

NRS = Normal rabbit serum
ATS = Rabbit anti-mouse thymocyte serum

Reprinted with permission from the Williams and Wilkins Co.,
Maryland. (31).

TABLE VII

AGE-DEPENDENT LOSS IN NZB/w MICE OF
ATS-INDUCED ENHANCEMENT OF THE ANTIBODY
RESPONSE TO rI·rC (100 µg)

Age (Months)	Treatment		ABC to rI·rC (µg/ml)	
	rI·rC	ATS	5 day	8 day
2	−	−	0.6	0.4
	+	−	2.1	0.5
	+	+	3.9	2.1
5	−	−	3.6	3.0
	+	−	4.2	3.6
	+	+	4.8	3.9
6	−	−	7.0	ND
	+	−	7.2	ND
	+	+	7.9	ND

Reprinted with permission from the Williams and Wilkins Co., Maryland. (31).

ATS-INDUCED ENHANCEMENT OF THE 5 DAY
ANTIBODY RESPONSE TO 100 µg rI·rC IN
6 MONTH OLD FEMALE MICE

Strain	Treatment		ABC to rI·rC
	rI·rC	ATS	
BALB/c	−	−	< 1.0
	+	−	7.4
	+	+	16.7
CDF₁	−	−	2.5
	+	−	7.1
	+	+	18.1
NZB/w	−	−	7.0
	+	−	7.2
	+	+	7.9

Reprinted with permission from the Williams and Wilkins Co., Maryland. (31).

regulatory function. The study was complicated by the spontaneous production of antibodies to RNA. This was circum-
vented by studying the response to SSSIII to which NZB mice
do not spontaneously produce antibodies (35). We found an
age associated increase in the antibody response to immunization with SSSIII. The increased response of older NZB mice
was reduced by syngeneic thymocytes from 4 week old donors
(35). Syngeneic thymocytes were also able to suppress the
high GVH response of spleen cells from 5 month old NZB/NZW
mice (36). The GVH studies have recently been extended (37).
It appears that GVH activity of NZB/NZW spleen cells increases in the first 6 months of life (apparently due to a loss of
suppressor cells) followed by a decline in GVH (Figure VII).

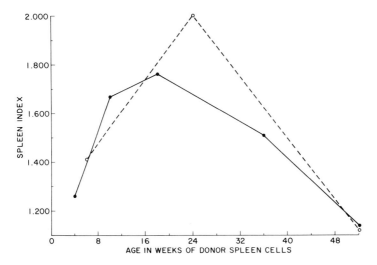

Fig. VII. GVH response, measured as spleen index 9 days
after injection of newborn C3H/HeJ mice, induced by 5 X 10[6]
spleen cells from NZB/NZW female mice of varying ages. The
dashed and solid lines represent 2 different series of experiments conducted one year apart. Reprinted with permission
from the Williams and Wilkins Co., Maryland.(37).

The decline in GVH appears to be related to a loss of helper
cells perhaps caused by the production of NTA (29,38). Particular attention was paid to the early loss of suppressor
cells. Between 4 and 16 weeks of age there was a gradual
decline in the ability of 1 X 10[6] thymocytes to suppress the
GVH capacity of 5 X 10[6] spleen cells from 4½ month old

NZB/NZW mice (Table IX). The degree of suppression was not
significant when the thymocytes were obtained from donors
older than 8 weeks of age (37). It appears from these

TABLE IX

GVH response of NZB/NZW spleen cells: suppression by 1
month thymocytes but not 4 month thymocytes in combination
with 4½ month spleen cells and synergy in combination with
12 month spleen cells.

| Donor Cell Population(s) | | Mean Spleen |
Thymocytes (1×10^6)	Spleen Cells (5×10^6)	Index
1 month	-	1.00
2 month	-	1.04
3 month	-	1.11
4 month	-	1.12
-	4½ month	1.75[c]
1 month	4½ month	1.29[a]
2 month	4½ month	1.34[b]
3 month	4½ month	1.58[c]
4 month	4½ month	1.71[c]
-	12 month	1.19
1 month	12 month	1.49[d]
4 month	12 month	1.51[d]

[a] $p < 0.01$ compared with 4½ month spleen cells alone,
   Student's t-test.
[b] $p < 0.05$ compared with 4½ month spleen cells alone,
   Student's t-test.
[c] not significantly different
[d] $p < 0.05$ compared with 12 month spleen cells alone,
   Student's t-test.

Reprinted with permission from the Williams and Wilkins Co.,
Maryland. (37).

experiments that with age New Zealand mice lose normal thymic regulatory or suppressor function. The importance of
this in their naturally occurring disease is illustrated in
Table X. Neonatal thymectomy led to accelerated anti-DNA
production (22). This could be prevented by grafting a syngeneic 2 week old thymus, thereby restoring thymic suppressor
function. Thymic grafts from 10 week old syngeneic donors
were ineffective, suggesting that by that age normal regula-

TABLE X
EFFECT OF THYMECTOMY AND THYMIC GRAFTS ON
ANTI-DNA ANTIBODY FORMATION IN NZB/NZW MICE

Treatment	Thymic Graft	Mean % DNA Bound	
		4 Months	5 Months
Sham	None	25.7	48.6
Thymectomy	None	42.8	69.4
Thymectomy	2 Week	21.4	50.4
Thymectomy	10 Week	41.0	67.1

Reprinted with permission from Harper & Row, New York. (30).

tory function had already been lost. In the absence of normal thymic regulatory functions New Zealand mice might be subject to excessive antibody responses to a variety of antigens including protein, nucleic acid, erythrocyte and leukocyte antigens. This would allow for a mechanism for loss of tolerance to a variety of self and foreign antigens as well as Gross viral antigens. The antibody responses to all of these substances could lead to immune complex disease characterized by several antigen-antibody systems. A role for thymic hormone as a mediator of regulatory function is an unproved but likely possibility (39,40). Whether the antithymocyte antibody of New Zealand mice is just one more autoantibody following loss of regulatory function or, in fact, is responsible for loss of regulatory cells will be a difficult problem to solve. It is possible that viral infection of the thymus plays a role in the early loss of normal thymic function in NZB/NZW mice. Nevertheless, the relative roles of genetic and viral factors in producing the loss of normal regulatory function remain to be determined.

The studies to date suggest three obvious therapeutic approaches to "autoimmunity" in New Zealand mice. The first is to non-specifically reduce immune responses. This can be accomplished with immunosuppressive drugs and can be quite effective. The second is to attempt to restore normal immune regulatory function. Administering thymic regulatory cells to NZB mice has markedly reduced the anti-erythrocyte antibodies (Figure VIII)(41). A less dramatic reduction in immune

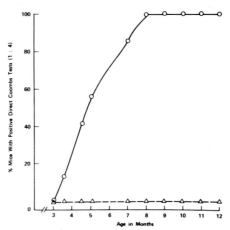

SUPPRESSED COOMBS TEST IN
NZB MICE TREATED WITH SYNGENEIC
YOUNG THYMOCYTES (Δ--Δ)

Figure VIII. NZB mice were treated from 4 weeks of age every fortnight with 50 X 10^6 thymocytes from NZB donors 2 weeks of age (Δ-----Δ) or with medium alone (o———o). (41).

---

complex disease has been achieved in NZB/NZW mice (42). The third, based upon the assumption that New Zealand mice harbor a unique virus which is solely responsible for disease, would be to treat the infection. However, it is possible that treatment after the onset of clinical disease might be too late to reverse the consequences of infection. Similar approaches are applicable to patients with SLE with some modifications. Suppressor cells could not be given from allogeneic donors; however, it is possible that a suppressor substance or thymic hormone might be successfully administered.

In summary, we have learned that known viral infections contracted when the host is immunologically incompetent can lead to chronic viremia. Antibody is produced which is inadequate to eliminate the virus from the circulation but which in combination with virus is deposited in the kidney. Whether or not clinical renal disease occurs depends upon 1) the particular virus and 2) the genetic susceptibility of the host. The spontaneously occurring autoimmune disease of New Zealand mice is associated with renal deposition of several antigen-antibody complexes; although Gross virus-antibody complexes are found in the kidney, nuclear antibody-antigen complexes are also present in greatest quantity. Evidence is presented to support the concept of thymic regulatory function. In New Zealand mice such regulatory function appears to be lost early in life. Immunologic abnormalities follow characterized by loss of tolerance to "self" and certain foreign protein, erythrocyte and nucleic acid antigens. These abnormalities lead to excessive antibody responses to the antigens thereby contributing to immune complex formation.

REFERENCES

1. Steinberg, A.D., Pincus, T. and Talal, N. (1969). J. Immunol. 102: 788.
2. Steinberg, A.D., Pincus, T. and Talal, N. (1971). Immunol. 20: 523.
3. Scher, I., Frantz, M. and Steinberg, A.D. (1973). J. Immunol. 110: 1396.
4. Steinberg, A.D., Baron, S. and Talal, N. (1969). Proc. Nat. Acad. Sci. 63: 1102.
5. Schur, P.H., Stollar, B.D., Steinberg, A.D. and Talal, N. (1971). Arthritis Rheum. 14: 342.
6. Talal, N., Steinberg, A.D. and Daley, G.G. (1971). J. Clin. Invest. 50: 1248.
7. Carpenter, D.F., Steinberg, A.D., Schur, P.H. and Talal, N. (1970). Lab. Invest. 23: 628.
8. Steinberg, A.D., Daley, G.G. and Talal, N. (1970). Science 167: 870.
9. Powell, D.E. and Steinberg, A.D. (1972). Clin. Exp. Immunol. 12: 419.
10. Talal, N., Steinberg, A.D., Jacobs, M.E., Chused, T.M. and Gazdar, A.F. (1971). J. Exp. Med. 34: 52s.
11. Lambert, P.H. and Dixon, F.J. (1968). J. Exp. Med. 127: 507.
12. Lambert, P.H. and Dixon, F.J. (1970). Clin. Exp. Immunol. 6: 829.
13. Mellors, R.C., Aoki, T. and Huebner, R.J. (1969). J. Exp. Med. 129: 1045.
14. Mellors, R.C., Shirai, T., Aoki, T.,Huebner, R.J. and Krawczynski, K. (1971). J. Exp. Med. 133: 113.
15. Oldstone, M.B. and Dixon, F.J. (1971). J. Exp. Med. 134: 32s.
16. Hoffsten, P.E. and Dixon, F.J. (1973). J. Exp. Med. 138: 887.
17. Cheema, A., Henson, J.B. and Gorham, J.R. (1972). Amer. J. Pathol. 66: 543.
18. Notkins, A.L. (1971). J. Exp. Med. 134: 41s.
19. Dixon, F.J., Oldstone, M.B. and Tonietti, G. (1971). J. Exp. Med. 134: 65s.
20. Oldstone, M.B.A. and Dixon, F.J. (1972). Science 175: 784.

21. Linder, E. and Edgington, T.S. (1972). Fed. Proc. 31: 766.
22. Koffler, D., Agnello, V., Thoburn, R. and Kunkel, H.G. (1971). J. Exp. Med. 134: 169s.
23. Baker, P.J. et.al. (1970). J. Immunol. 105: 1581.
24. Gershon, R.K., Cohen, P. et.al. (1972). J. Immunol. 108: 586.
25. Droege, W. (1971). Nature 234: 549.
26. Kerbel, R.S. and Eidinger, D. (1972). Europ. J. Immunol. 2: 114.
27. Okumura, K. and Tada, T. (1971). J. Immunol. 107: 1682.
28. Jacobson, E.B., et.al. (1972). J. Exp. Med. 135: 1163.
29. Shirai, T. and Mellors, R.C. (1971). Proc. Nat. Acad. Sci. 68: 1412.
30. Steinberg, A.D., Law, L.W. and Talal, N. (1970). Arthritis Rheum. 13: 369.
31. Chused, T.M., Steinberg, A.D. and Parker, L.M. (1973). J. Immunol. 111: 52.
32. Parker, L.M. and Steinberg, A.D. (1973). J. Immunol. 110: 742.
33. Weir, D.M., McBride, W. and Naysmith, J.D. (1968). Nature 219: 1276.
34. Staples, P.J. and Talal, N. (1969). J. Exp. Med. 129:123.
35. Barthold, D.R., Kysela, S. and Steinberg, A.D. (1974). J. Immunol. 112: 9.
36. Hardin, J.A., Chused, T.M. and Steinberg, A.D. (1973). J. Immunol. 111: 650.
37. Gerber, N.L., Hardin, J.A., Chused, T.M. and Steinberg, A.D. (1974). J. Immunol. 113: 1618.
38. Gelfand, M.C., Parker, L.M. and Steinberg, A.D. (1974). J. Immunol. 113: 1.
39. Bach, J-F., Dardenne, M. and Salomon, J-C. (1973). Clin. Exp. Immunol. 14: 247.
40. Dauphinee, M.J., Talal, N. et.al. (1974). Proc. Nat. Acad. Sci. 71: 2637.
41. Gershwin, M.E. and Steinberg, A.D. Clinical Immunol. and Immunopathol. In Press.
42. Kysela, S. and Steinberg, A.D. (1973). Clin. Immunol. and Immunopathol. 2: 133.

8

Immunoprophylaxis and Immunotherapy of Virus Infections

Stanley A. Plotkin

PATHOGENESIS OF VIRAL DISEASES

The methods for preventing viral diseases depend on the pathogenesis of the disease. On this basis, one can distinguish four kinds of viral diseases: First, there are those diseases in which the pathologic manifestations occur largely on the mucosal surface. The agents that come to mind immediately are the respiratory viruses, (although that term includes viruses which do spread beyond the mucosal surfaces).

The second, the archetype of viral disease, includes those agents which multiply on a mucosal surface, either the upper respiratory tract or the intestine, and then enter the bloodstream in a cell-free state; that is, free in the serum. During the viremia there is involvement of <u>viscera</u> and eventually clinical symptoms of illness. Poliomyelitis is a classic case of this phenomenon in which the virus spreads to the central nervous system. There are many other examples, including Fenner's well-described mousepox model (1). Measles, mumps, infectious hepatitis, rubella, and many other viruses are in this category.

The third group consists of the arboviruses and is more or less similar to the second, except for one important difference: the viruses are inoculated directly into the bloodstream by insects. From the bloodstream they often spread to the central nervous system.

Finally, there is a group in which the pathogenesis is not completely understood, but in which the initial event occurs on the mucosal surfaces, and then spreads in a cell-associated manner to other organs. This group includes the herpes viruses. Although there may be some viremia involved in herpes simplex infection, the more important fact is that it ascends the nerve tracts to the nerve cells in the ganglia. Rabies belongs to this group, also, since the virus ascends the nerve tract through the cellular appendages called axons.

Protective mechanisms on the mucosal surfaces differ from those in the bloodstream. Humoral antibodies are capable of neutralizing virus in the bloodstream, but they have little or no effect on neutralizing viruses on the mucosal surfaces. IgA secretory antibodies are needed for mucosal protection. Taking the varying pathogenic and immune response mechanisms into account, we can then look at the means of prophylaxis: killed and live virus vaccines.

KILLED VIRUS VACCINES: ADVANTAGES

Killed virus vaccines have been, until recently, made from whole virions; that is, the entire virion is inactivated and a large number of dead viruses are administered by injection. These vaccines work basically because the most important protective antigens are on the surface of virus particles. However, the fact that one has to inactivate an infectious virion introduces a number of safety problems, as was demonstrated in the "Cutter incident" in which the inactivation of certain batches of poliovirus was incomplete.

Recently it has been possible to break up the virion of influenza and other viruses and to isolate the protective antigens, thus increasing the safety factor and effectiveness. Therefore, an advantage of killed vaccines, if inactivated correctly, is that there is no danger of causing the disease you mean to prevent.

KILLED VIRUS VACCINES: DISADVANTAGES

There are several disadvantages in the use of killed vaccines. One is that no matter how powerful an antigen, and that includes tetanus toxoid, it is extremely difficult to immunize an individual with one injection of a killed antigen. With killed vaccines the antigen is incapable of repli-

cating and therefore repeated injections are necessary to
provoke a continued antibody response.

A second disadvantage is that, although killed antigens
produce humoral antibodies, they do not, by and large, produce antibodies on the mucosal surfaces. A third disadvantage
is if a killed antigen is insufficiently potent, it may sen-
sitize without protecting. Although killed measles vaccine
did protect at first, the humoral antibody response disap-
peared after a number of years leaving behind a cellular
hypersensitivity. This could be demonstrated by a marked response to skin test with measles antigen indicating mobiliza-
tion of sensitized lymphocytes. When the vaccinee was later
exposed to wild measles virus, he developed a case of measles
which was more severe than natural measles. Fortunately, few
recipients died. Those that did had mononuclear exudates in
their lungs. Humoral antibodies could be detected within a
week of exposure to measles antigen. This rise indicated a
definite booster response, but one which was too late to protect the individuals.

One could postulate that no humoral antibodies blocked the
virus from invading the mucosa, getting into the bloodstream
and being transported to organs containing sensizited lymphocytes in the lungs or in the reticuloendothelial system.
There the virus and the cellular antibody produce a pathologic
reaction. It is this phenomenon rather than an extensive
multiplication of measles virus that was important pathoge-
netically. Although the killed virus vaccinees had a severe
disease, they did not excrete more virus than children with
regular measles.

Some investigators believe that the hypersensitivity reaction was not to the measles antigen, but to something else.
The killed measles vaccine contained alum, and there are
those who argue that without the adjuvant the sensitizing
phenomenon wouldn't have occurred at all.

A group of live measles vaccinees was discovered recently
that makes an interesting comparison. A small percentage of
these vaccinees developed antibodies and lost them, but after
exposure to wild measles they had a normal immune response
and a mild disease. So, after reinfection, they did not show
cellular hypersensitivity, although they had also lost humoral antibody.

LIVE VACCINE - SELECTION

Live vaccines differ from killed vaccines in many ways.
First of all, the selection of attenuated variants, (which is
what is involved when you prepare a live vaccine), is essen-

tially the selection of a pre-existing particle from the original population. For example, some years ago in developing attenuated polio strains, we took a wild virus and passed it at low temperatures so that it would grow at 23°C and not at 40°C. At the same time, we plaqued the original virus and picked a number of plaques and passed them individually. With passage of the general population we found the gradual development of ability to grow at 23°C and a converse inability to grow at 40°C. With the passage of single plaque populations we found that one particular plaque showed a sudden change after the third passage from an inability to grow at 23°C to a rather striking ability to grow at this temperature. The implication here is that one can select by passage that part of the original population that does what one determines is a good thing for it to do and thus allow that genetic variant to become predominant. One takes a single property which, in the case of polio is growth at low temperatures, and hopes that it correlates with other useful biologic properties, for example, failure to produce viremia. Of course, a number of different methods are used to produce attenuation including recently, induction of temperature sensitive mutants.

Advantages

One advantage of vaccination with attenuated virus is that it mimics natural infection more closely than does killed virus. As a result live vaccines usually restrict mucosal infection by wild virus by triggering an IgA response. Table 1 shows, for example, the administration of attenuated polio

TABLE 1

Intestinal Infection by Attenuated Type 1 Polioviruses in Immune and Susceptible Individuals

	Chat Strain		LSC-2ab Strain	
Immune Status	No. of Subjects	Mean Duration of Fecal Virus Excretion (days)	No. of Subjects	Mean Duration of Fecal Virus Excretion (days)
Nonimmunes	56	24	30	20
Live virus vaccinees	34	2	33	5
Natural immunes	7	1	69	4

virus to people who had not been immunized before, to people who had had live vaccine before, and to people who had had polio infection. The mean duration of viral excretion was 24 days in susceptible individuals, 2 days in live virus vaccinees, and 1 day in natural immunes. When live polio virus was given to a killed virus vaccinated group, the mean duration of excretion was very similar to that in non-immunes.

Still another advantage of live vaccines is persistence of immunity. Humoral immunity seems to last indefinitely, and secretory antibody either persists or is rapidly recalled to provide immunity on challenge years later. The explanation for this is that live virus replication presents the organism with a lot more antigen than does the killed virus. All of the antigens of the virus are created in vivo and the host has a chance to respond to many structural components; with killed vaccine one is only immunizing against certain surface antigens. Of course, even immunity after natural infection, at least as measured by antibody levels, does decline with time. In most natural infections, also, if one looks at the median titers of antibody in people of various ages, the highest titers are in children. The idea has been proposed that the reason for the long persistence of viral immunity after natural infection or after live virus vaccines is that the virus itself persists in some latent form. An example of persistence is subacute sclerosing panencephalitis (SSPE) wherein the wild measles virus does, in fact, persist in the brain. However, there is no conclusive evidence that attenuated measles vaccine virus can persist, also.

For one group of viruses, there is no doubt that the viruses do persist. This is the herpes virus group, including herpes simplex, cytomegalovirus, and varicella zoster. In herpes there is an ascending infection up the nerve from the skin. The virus then enters the dorsal ganglia and becomes latent and inaccessible to antibody. In mice and in man also, if one removes the trigeminal ganglia and explants the ganglia in culture, eventually herpes simplex virus will grow. Presumably in vivo the virus comes back down the nerve to the skin to cause a recurrence. It is certain that the herpes viruses do not reside in the skin. In other words, if one removes the skin one cannot prevent recurrences. One can prevent them, however, by cutting the nerve.

No defect in humoral, secretory or cellular immunity has yet been discovered that explains the phenomenon of recurrence. During an herpetic recurrence the virus spreads from cell to cell despite the presence of antibody. There are well-known clinical stimuli for reactivation, like menstruation, and ultraviolet exposure, but the host factors that are operative have yet to be described. There is also no tenable explanation at the moment for why the herpetic lesion does regress. Interferon response or migration of immune cells into the lesion may be part of the answer. Antigenic differences among herpes viruses appear to be insufficient to explain recurrences since people who have recurrences have an excess of antibody. There are strain variations, but these have been defined with sensitive tests and with strains that have been passaged in the laboratory many times, and there appears to be no clinical significance to these strain variations.

Disadvantages

The first disadvantage of live vaccine is the safety factor. In biology there is bound to be someone at the end of the bell-shaped population curve who is susceptible to even the attenuated form of a disease. In him you may cause the disease that you're trying to prevent. For example, the Type 3 Sabin polio vaccine does have an ability to produce poliomyelitis in a small percentage of vaccinees, particularly in adults.

The second problem is the maintenance of the right level of attenuation. There are many examples: mumps, live influenza and rubella. Merck Sharpe & Dohme developed 5 different passage levels of a rubella virus in duck embryo culture: the strain at level A produced rubella and was not useful as a vaccine; at level B, it produced a fairly high rate of reaction; at level D the antibody response was poor; at level E, it failed to produce any antibody response in the majority of people. Level C was just right. This is the kind of test that must be done often with attenuated vaccines. An attenuated virus must replicate in the host. Some temperature sensitive viruses are useless as vaccines because they will not replicate at $37^{\circ}C$. Now there are exceptions to that rule; for example, the live high egg passage (HEP) rabies vaccine can be used in man as an antigen, but it doesn't replicate.

If one starts out with a wild polio virus at first passage level it may produce paralysis in monkeys injected with 10 TCD_{50}. With passage, it becomes less virulent until, by the 50th passage 10^6 TCD_{50} are required to produce paralysis. One has reduced its ability to cause polio by 100,000 times. So, if cne started with a wild virus capable of producing polio 50% of the time in man, in theory the risk would have been reduced to .0005%.

Ideally, attenuated polio strains do not cause viremia, and multiply only in the gut. However, there is evidence that on occasion viremia does occur. Because the strain is attenuated, the viremia may not necessarily lead to multiplication in the central nervous system.

Other problems that may come up with live viruses include interference by other agents either directly by the presence of that virus or indirectly, by interferon induction. Also, some attenuated viruses such as polio virus replicate on mucosal surfaces, are excreted, and can be spread to contacts. This has its benefits in terms of immunizing contacts, but it also has its risks in terms of causing disease in contacts, if reversion to virulence occurs. There is no doubt that reversion to virulent strains occurs in some vaccinees. This has been demonstrated quite clearly with polio vaccine. The virus that comes out of the patient is often more virulent than when it went in, and one can show that if stools are collected on each day one will find a gradual increase in virulence. However, if one takes this virus and injects it into monkeys, although it is clearly more virulent, it is still much less virulent than a wild polio virus. One experiment which was done in Russia took excreted attenuated polio virus and passed it ten times in man by taking the fecal virus, culturing it, and feeding the culture fluid. At the end of the ten passages there was still no disease and the virus was still less virulent than wild virus. So, apparently it takes quite a number of mutations to get back to the original state of virulence.

RESPONSES TO IMMUNIZATION

As stated before, vaccination with attenuated virus is supposed to mimic natural infection, but this is not always so. In the case of rubella virus, there are three attenuated strains and, of course, there's also wild rubella virus. There are many different ways of measuring rubella antibody. When one looks at the hemagglutination inhibition response, for example, one finds the natural virus producing distinctly higher levels of antibodies than the attenuated virus. Complement fixation shows the same sort of difference. In the case of precipitin antibodies there is the interesting observation that the natural infection produces two types of precipitins, or perhaps one should say that there are two identified antigens, theta and iota, and antibodies can be demonstrated to both antigens in natural infection. In attenuated infection, however, we see that the theta antigen (which corresponds to the hemagglutinin) does produce antibodies, but the iota antigen does not, except in the case of the RA27/3 strain which produces both antibodies (Table 2). There are also differences in the production of secretory antibody which probably depend on the extent of multiplication on the mucosa (3)(Table 3). After natural disease there are high levels of nasal antibody. After Cendehill

TABLE 2

Precipitin Responses to Rubella Vaccines
(Le Bouvier, 1969; Le Bouvier and Plotkin, 1971)

Vaccine Strain	Antibodies to Antigens Theta	Iota
HPV-77	16/20	5/20
Cendehill	15/15	1/15
RA 27/3*	33/33	32/33

* Subcutaneous and Intranasal

TABLE 3
Serum and Nasal Antibody Titers Two Months
After Natural Infection or Vaccination
(ogra et al, 1971)

Virus	Serum Antibody No. Pos./Total	GMT-HAI	Nasal Antibody No.Pos./Total	GMT-RAI
Natural	25/25	725	24/25	23
HPV-77-DK	30/30	170	0/30	<1
RA27/3-IN	15/15	209	13/15	8
RA27/3-SC	5/5	80	2/5	2

vaccination, although viral replication occurs in the naso-
pharynx, mucosal antibody does not occur. The RA27/3 intro-
duced intranasally does produce nasal antibody, but the same
vaccine given subcutaneously gives lower levels. The importance of this observation is shown in Table 4. If one challenges someone who has had natural rubella with either the
Cendehill subcutaneously, RA27/3 subcutaneously, or the
RA27/3 vaccine intranasally, no antibody boost occurs. The
same is true for those who had previously received the intranasal vaccine, whereas those who had received Cendehill live
vaccine parenterally, which elicited no nasal antibody, were
capable of being reinfected. So, in this case, it is not
just a black and white distinction between killed and live
vaccines. There are differences between live vaccines in the
extent of the protection afforded which depends upon the

TABLE 4

BOOSTER VACCINATION BY REINFECTION OF PREVIOUSLY
VACCINATED INDIVIDUALS

BOOSTER	PREVIOUS IMMUNIZATION		
	NATURAL	RA27/3-IN	CENDEHILL
CENDEHILL	0/10	0/10	0/10
RA27/3-SC	0/10	2/10	1/8
RA27/3-IN	1/10	1/10	7/10
PLACEBO	0/10	0/10	0/10

types of antibodies being produced.

If antibody is produced, the lymphocytes must be capable of responding to a particular antigen, and therefore are themselves sensitized. There are many pieces of evidence for cellular immunity in viral diseases. Vaccinia is a classical example of the situation in which rare people who produce humoral antibodies are nevertheless unable to contain a vaccination; that is, the vaccine lesion continues to spread and can, in fact, kill the individual if allowed to go on. Deficiency in "cellular immunity" is the most obvious explanation. Patients with Bruton's agammaglobulinemia, that is, who do not produce circulatory antibody, but are capable of responding with cellular hypersensitivity, can cope with smallpox or measles vaccines, whereas individuals who have cellular immune defects develop vaccinia gangrenosa or measles giant cell pneumonia, which are usually fatal.

Often with respiratory viruses mucosal antibody is more important than the humoral antibody in protecting against the disease. Table 5 shows the levels of serum and mucosal antibodies in people who were challenged with parainfluenza Type 1. The group with the maximum protection was the one that had both high serum and nasal antibodies, but the group with high nasal antibody and little serum antibody was also very well protected. This phenomenon has been demonstrated with many different viruses. In the case of polio there is no doubt that the reason why people who receive live virus get protection from challenge is that there's IgA secretory antibody in the gut. This was demonstrated very nicely by Ogra

TABLE 5

IMPORTANCE OF ANTIBODIES IN THE NASAL
SECRETIONS IN THE PREVENTION OF INFECTION WITH
PARAINFLUENZA TYPE 1 VIRUS

Neutralizing antibody in nasal secretions	Neutralizing antibody in serum	
	Low	High
Low	10/13	3/4
High	1/9	0/8

who took infants with colostomies and inoculated virus directly into the colon and showed that secretory antibody developed
only in the colon and did not develop elsewhere. Humoral
antibody also developed. So, the process of direct viral multiplication produces local secretory antibody and generalized
serum antibody. Despite the secretory antibody response to
live polio virus vaccination virus excretion may go on for
several weeks, perhaps longer. During that time the quantity
of virus present in the gut is apparently sufficiently in
excess so that whatever secretory antibody has been formed
does not eliminate it.

PASSIVE PROTECTION

Gammaglobulin, by providing artificial antibody, is another
means of prophylaxis, but gammaglobulin is only useful in
diseases where viremia is important as, for example, polio,
measles, and rubella. Table 6 shows the results of rubella

TABLE 6

EFFECT OF GAMMAGLOBULIN ON RUBELLA

Group	Rash	Day on Which Rash Appeared	Virus in Pharynx	Virus in Blood	Antibody Response
Controls	6/6	12	6/6	5/6	6/6
Gammaglobulin 24 hrs. post infection	0/6	--	4/6	0/6	4/6

studies. When seronegative individuals were given live rubella virus, all 6 had clinical rubella and virus in the pharynx within an incubation period of 12 days and 5 out of 6 had virus in the blood. All later developed antibodies. Another group of 6 seronegatives received ordinary gammaglobulin 24 hours after infection. The gammaglobulin came from pools of blood donors who have natural antibodies to rubella, since rubella is a ubiquitous infection. None of them developed a rash, but 4 of the gammaglobulin group did show infection in the pharynx. Thus, humoral antibody had little effect on pharyngeal infection. However, none of the gammaglobulin-treated group had viremia. This illustrates the value of gammaglobulin in preventing viremia, but it is only useful when the prevention of viremia prevents disease.

This work was supported by a grant from the Smith, Kline and French Laboratories.

REFERENCES

1. Fenner, F. (1950). In: The Pathogenesis and Pathology of Viral Diseases (Kidd, J.G., ed.), p. 99, Columbia University Press, New York.
2. Hilleman, M.R. (1969). Science 164: 506.
3. Ogra, P.L. et.al. (1971). New Eng. J. Med. 285: 1333.

9

Vaccines of the Future: Immunogenicity of Viral Components

Frantisek Sokol

Virologists working in the field of immunity against viral
infections turn to molecular biologists for help usually for
two reasons. First, they want the viral antigen(s) which is
(are) capable of eliciting the formation of virus neutralizing antibodies to be identified and characterized. Second,
they want to prepare a subunit vaccine. The first seems to
be a trivial task since simple methods are available for
determining the overall protein composition of a virus and
for localizing structural proteins within the virion. The
analytical part of the problem is usually accomplished by
dissociating the protein moiety of the virus into polypeptides which are subsequently fractionated on the basis of
differences in molecular size, net charge, solubility, etc.
Localization of the viral proteins within the virion is
usually determined by controlled degradation of the virus
into subviral structures followed by analysis of the polypep-
tide composition of the solubilized fraction and the residual sub-virion structure. The surface antigens of a virus
can be identified by tagging them with exogenous compounds
such as isotopically labeled substances. Of course, the
tagging procedure must not disintegrate the virion. This is
particularly important since antigens localized on the surface of the infectious entity (virus or subviral infectious
core) are the ones which induce neutralizing antibody formation in the immunized organism. The final proof in identifying antigens which induce immunity against viral diseases is

---

*The editors wish to mark with sorrow the death of Dr.
Frantisek Sokol who succumbed to a myocardial infarction
shortly after writing his chapter.

achieved by isolating their surface proteins in pure form and
by assaying of their ability to elicit virus neutralizing
antibody formation. As it turns out not all surface antigens
can elicit synthesis of virus neutralizing antibodies. Thus
antibodies against neuraminidase of influenza virions failed
to neutralize the infectivity of the virus, although it is
known that this enzyme is localized on the surface of the
virus particles. However, antibodies against the enzyme were
able to block the egress of influenza virions from the infected cells, resulting in suppression of spreading of the
infection (1,2,3). No matter how trivial this first task
might sound, it is often a tedious one, the interpretation
of the seemingly simple experiments leading to many contro-
versies and ambiguities (4). There are many reasons for
these difficulties: the impurity of the obtained viral fractions, the decreased immunogenicity of dissociated viral components in comparison with that of intact virions, the un-
avoidable destruction of certain antigenic determinants by
dissociation of the virus (mainly those involving amino acid
residues from two or several distinct polypeptides), extensive denaturation of the viral components by the dissociating
agents and by the fractionation procedures and formation of
new antigenic determinants which were not present in the
virions. Despite these difficulties the surface antigens
capable of binding virus neutralizing antibodies and inducing their formation in immunized animals have been identified
and characterized in many viruses (4).

More frequently the biochemist is asked to work out a procedure for preparation of a "subunit" vaccine, a vaccine containing the solubilized, type-specific viral surface antigen.
Depending on the degree of purity of the subunit vaccine, the
group-specific (core) viral antigens might be present or ab-
sent from the preparation. The specific protective activity
of the subunit vaccine is much lower than that of a live virus vaccine and even lower than that of inactivated virion
vaccine. Not only do the virions from the live vaccine replicate in the vaccinated individual and amplify the immune response, but also the immunogenicity of the virion vaccines is
higher due to the enormous difference in the molecular weight
of the antigens in the virion and subunit preparations, respectively. In addition, it will be recalled that certain
antigenic determinants of intact virions are not present in
subunit vaccine.

The demand for such a product is justified, however, by
the need for a vaccine devoid of pyrogens or substances
capable of eliciting the release of pyrogens and of viral
nucleic acid. Pyrogenicity of virions is markedly decreased

during the preparation of the subunit vaccines by treatment with lipid solvents or detergents (5,6). The viral nucleic acids, DNA directly and RNA after transcription into a complementary DNA, are potentially capable of becoming integrated into the cellular genome. In this way, the presence of the viral genome in the cell can escape control by immunity or interferon action. Under suitable conditions the viral genome can be excised and replicated in the host, which might lead to additional integration of the viral nucleic acid into the cellular DNA. The accumulative integration of a goreign nucleic acid may result in increasing metabolic disorders such as those seen in neoplasia or slow virus disease. One should stress, however, that there is no evidence for such harmful effects in live or inactivated virion vaccines. The above reasoning represents perhaps, the "overconcerned" rationale of advocates of nucleic acid-free virus vaccines. This concern is not without justification since it has been shown that oncogenic viruses inactivated by radiation may exhibit an even higher tumorigenicity or ability to transform cells in vitro than untreated virions (7).

There are two possible sources of viral subunits. They can be derived from crude or purified virion preparations which have been partially dissociated by nonionic or weak ionic detergents, by exposure to high salt environment, heating, organic solvents or exposure to alkaline environment (4, 8). Once the protein moiety of the virus has been dissociated, the envelope or coat (surface) antigens can be separated from the core components and the viral nucleic acid by a variety of fractionation techniques. As an example, the aggregated envelope glycoproteins of dissociated influenza virus or paramyxoviruses which contain hemagglutinating and neuraminidase activity, can be separated from other viral components, including the viral RNA, by selective adsorption onto and elution from erythrocytes (9). If just the removal of the viral nucleic acids is requested, they can be degraded by treatment with minute amounts of nucleases of appropriately dissociated virus preparation, containing free, not encapsidated viral RNA or DNA.

Another rich source of solubilized viral antigens is the infected cell and tissue culture fluid freed of virus particles, i.e., the supernatant fluid obtained after high speed centrifugation of disrupted host cells or of infectious tissue culture fluid.

The "soluble antigens" probably represent "surplus" products of infection. These are viral components which were not assembled into virions, although a portion of sub-viral components may be formed also by degradation of virus particles. One has to realize that a crude soluble antigen

131

vaccine will always contain more host cell components than crude virion or virion-derived vaccines. It will also be more difficult, if not impossible, to free a soluble antigen vaccine from the bulk of the host cell components than a corresponding virion vaccine. The possibility of preparing vaccines from infected cell homogenates or from the soluble fraction of infectious tissue culture fluids remains attractive only because of the richness of these sources in viral antigens. Clearly, infected cells synthesize a large excess of viral antigens which are not utilized for virion assembly.

I shall illustrate the general conclusion I made so far by a concrete example. For many years my colleagues and I have been involved in attempts to improve the existing vaccines against rabies and to elucidate the antigenic structure of rabies virus. Rabies virus is an RNA containing enveloped virus, the viral envelope consisting of proteins, glycoproteins, and lipids. The virus can be grown in relatively high yields in hamster kidney, monkey kidney or human diploid cell cultures. Three out of the 4 major protein components were found to be constituents of the viral envelope: the spike glycoprotein (emerging from the membrane) (G) and 2 membrane proteins (Ml and M2). The viral RNA is intimately associated with core phosphoprotein molecules (N protein) to form the nucleocapsid of the virus (10,11,12). When purified virus preparations are treated with deoxycholate, a weak ionic detergent, in isotonoic environment, the whole viral envelope (lipids, G protein, Ml and M2 proteins) are solubilized and the remaining subviral structure, the filamentous nucleocapsid composed of all the viral RNA and about 1700 molecules of N phosphoprotein (11), can be separated from the solubilized envelope components by velocity centrifugation (10) (Figure 1). After removal of the deoxycholate by dialysis or gel filtration, the solubilized fraction can be utilized as a subunit vaccine. Treatment of purified virions with a nonionic detergent, such as Nonidet P-40 (13,14) in isotonic or hypotonic environments results in preferential solubilization of viral lipids and the G protein. The remaining "skeleton" particles, composed of all the viral RNA, N phosphoprotein and Ml and M2 membrane proteins can be separated from the G protein by velocity centrifugation. Comparison of the immunogenicity of viral fractions, which were obtained from virions degraded by these two methods, has shown that the G protein of rabies virus is the only antigen capable of eliciting virus neutralizing antibody formation, of binding these antibodies and of protecting immunized animals against subsequent challenge by rabies virus (15). Also, the envelope glycoprotein is the component of

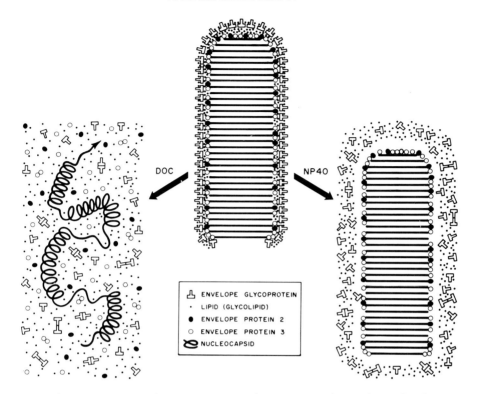

Fig. 1. Schematic representation of partial dissociation of rabies virions by sodium deoxycholate or Nonidet P-40. Reprinted with permission from The Williams & Wilkins Co., Maryland.

the virus which binds to the surface receptors of the cells and initiates the entry of the virions into the host. Thus, subunit vaccines can be prepared from rabies virions treated either with deoxycholate or a nonionic detergent(16). After removal from the preparation of the viral core and of the detergent the subunit vaccine is ready to be used. As expected, however, the specific immunogenicity or specific protective activity of such vaccines is markedly lower than that of virion vaccines (15) for reasons which have already been explained. It can presumably be improved by aggregation of the antigen. This has been shown to be the case with the envelope glycoproteins of influenza virus which give rise to neutralizing antibody formation (17).

One important activity of rabies virion vaccines is, how-ever, completely missing from subunit vaccines. Both live and inactivated rabies virions are good inducers of interfer-on which contributes to the protective activity of the vaccine preparation (18). Solubilized protein components of the virus devoid of viral RNA are not interferon inducers.

Infectious tissue culture fluids freed of rabies virions by high-speed centrifugation, selective precipitation or ultrafiltration elicit virus neutralizing antibody formation in inoculated animals (19,20,21). The protective activity of such preparations rests in the solubilized G protein molecules rather than in the residual virions. The immunogenicity and the protective activity of these soluble-antigens can be improved markedly when the tissue culture fluid is freed of virions by precipitation with zinc acetate. Zinc acetate causes the aggregation of the soluble antigens. Since infection with rabies virus does not cause lysis of the host cells, the infectious tissue culture fluid is relatively little contaminated with cellular components. Rabies virus can be grown in high yield utilizing tissue culture media devoid of serum. Thus, it would not be too tedious to work out procedures for concentration and purification of the viral glycoprotein from this source.

This investigation was supported by U.S. Public Health Research Grants ROI-CA10594 and CA-10815 from the National Cancer Institute and AI-09706 from the National Institute of Allergy and Infectious Diseases; by Grant SP-121964 from the Commonwealth of Pennsylvania, Department of Health, and by funds from the World Health Organization.

REFERENCES

1. Compans, R.W., Dimmock, N.J. and Meier-Ewert, H. (1969). J. Virol. 4: 528.
2. Kilbourne, E.D., Laver, W.G., Schulman, J.L. and Webster, R.G. (1968). J. Virol. 2: 281.
3. Seto, J.T. and Rott, R. (1966). Virology 30: 731.
4. Neurath, A.R. and Rubin, B.A. (1971). In: Monographs in Virology, Vol. 4. (Melnick, J.L., ed.). S. Karger, Basel.
5. Davenport, F.M., Henessy, A.V., Brandon, F.M., Webster, R.G. et.al. (1964). J. Lab. Clin. Med. 63: 5.
6. Duxbury, A.E., Hampson, A.W. and Sievers, J.G.M. (1968). J. Immunol. 101: 62.
7. Defendi, V. and Jensen, F. (1967). Science 157: 703.
8. Sokol, F. (1971). In: Recent Advances in Microbiology, Xth Int. Congr. Microbiol. (Pérez-Miravete, A. and Peláéz, D., eds.), Mexico City.

9. Sokol, F., Blaškovič, D., and Križanová-Laučiková, O. (1961). Nature (London) 190: 834.

10. Sokol, F., Schlumberger, H.D., Wiktor, T.J., et.al.(1969). Virology 38: 651.

11. Sokol, F., Stanček, D., and Koprowski, H. (1971). J. Virol 7: 241.

12. Sokol, F. and Clark, H F. (1973). Virology 52 : 246.

13. György, E., Sheehan, M.C., and Sokol, F. (1971). J. Virol. 8: 649.

14. Kelley, J.M., Emerson, S.U. and Wagner, R.R. (1972). J. Virol. 10: 1231.

15. Wiktor, T.J., György, E., Schlumberger, H.D. et.al.(1973). J. Immunol. 110: 269.

16. Neurath, A.R., Vernon, S.K., Dobkin, M.B. and Rubin, B.A. (1972). J. Gen. Virol. 14: 33.

17. Laver, W.G. and Valentine, R.C. (1969). Virology 38: 105.

18. Wiktor, T.J., Postic, B., Ho, M. and Koprowski, H. (1972). J. Inf. Dis. 126: 408.

19. Crick, J. and Brown, F. (1969). Nature (London) 222: 92.

20. Wiktor, T.J., Sokol, F., Kuwert, E. and Koprowski, H. (1969). Proc. Soc. Exp. Biol. Med. 131: 799.

21. Schlumberger, H.D., Wiktor, T.J. and Koprowski, H. (1970). J. Immunol. 105: 291.

AUTHOR INDEX

SUBJECT INDEX

A 5
B 6
C 7
D 8
E 9
F 0
G 1
H 2
I 3
J 4